DEAR FUTURE
MAMA

DEAR FUTURE
MAMA

A TMI Guide to Pregnancy, Birth, and
New Motherhood from Your Bestie

Meghan Trainor

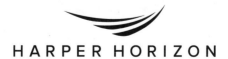

HARPER HORIZON

For Riley, who made me a mom.
For my mom, who showed me how it's done.
And for Daryl, who makes my life complete.

CONTENTS

PART 3: TRIMESTER THREE

PART 4: TRIMESTER FOUR

DEAR FUTURE MAMA

Dear Future Mama,

I'm full-on obsessed with pregnancy in all its weird, painful, messy glory. I'm the friend (wanna be friends?) who wants to know when and how you started trying, what multivitamin you're on, when you got the positive test, when you felt your first kick . . . and how it felt to poop for the first time after baby. It doesn't matter how crazy you were in college or how many things you've already crossed off your bucket list—this experience is going to be the wildest thing you've ever done. Your body is doing amazing, beautiful, and very strange things right now. For example: giving you intense heartburn when all you've eaten is one plain, tasteless cracker, or sending shooting pain from your hip to your leg, or making your hair extra luscious but also giving you terrible acne. Maybe your gums are bleeding, or your hips hurt, or for some reason only your right armpit is sweating. While you sleep, or eat, or go to work, your entire body is basically 3D-printing a human being.

    I spent my entire pregnancy trying to get all the information I could possibly get, mostly by watching hours of YouTube—so much that my husband, Daryl, threatened to delete the app from all my devices. I couldn't help it; I was fascinated by what I was experiencing, and as the first of my friends to be pregnant, nobody around me but my mom, my aunts, and strangers on the internet knew what I was going through. And because my mom and my aunts kept saying, "Meghan, that was decades ago, you think I remember?" moms on YouTube became my imaginary besties.

My friends couldn't relate to aching boobs or weird dreams or feeling like a baby was trying to escape through my ribs, but they heard about it anyway because they're good friends and because I was going to tell them whether they liked it or not. Sure, they thought I was crazy sometimes (and cringed when I shared the grosser details), but they also told me that everything I shared with them helped them feel a lot less nervous about having their own babies someday.

That's exactly what I hope this book does for you! Pregnancy can be exciting and scary, confusing and a little lonely, even when you're surrounded by love. I want to keep it real without freaking you out, make you laugh and shout *"OMG, same!"* I want to make sure you know the most important things every mama needs to know: that you're enough, that you're made for this, and that you are the perfect mama that this baby has been waiting for.

So read this book like it's just the two of us, hanging out talking about what the fuck is going on in our uteruses, because I gotchu, queen.

Love,

INTRODUCTION

I was twelve years old and absolutely not planning to witness my first birth *and* see my aunt's vagina, but sometimes these things just happen.

My mom's little sister, Lisa, is ten years younger than her and always felt more like my big sister than my aunt. She'd already been in labor with her first baby for hours, and my mom let me tag along to the hospital, where we planned to pass the time in the waiting room until my new cousin arrived.

Even as a kid, I knew that motherhood was my destiny. I grew up with more baby dolls than Barbie dolls, and I treated these dolls like they were actual babies with personalities and preferences. Even after I outgrew the baby dolls and started singing and writing my own music, I knew that what I wanted to be when I grew up was an international recording artist . . . and a mom. Blame my mom, Kelli—she's perfect, seriously. She's the most selfless person I know. My entire childhood, she made motherhood look *fun*, even when my brothers and I drove her crazy. I didn't want to be just any mom, I wanted to be a mom like *her*: the kind of mom who played hide-and-seek, who went trick-or-treating even when it was freezing cold, who told her kids to roll down the car windows and "scream it out" to let off steam, and who gave "lay-down time" to all three of her kids every single night, rubbing our backs for what felt like hours just so we could fall asleep feeling safe and loved.

I was in seventh grade and was as excited as anyone in our family about my aunt's new baby. I couldn't *wait* to meet him, but waiting is exactly what you do in the waiting room, and nobody knew how long it would take. When Lisa's husband—my uncle Burton—came out to see us, he looked exhausted. The contractions seemed to have stopped, he told us. Did we want to go in and say hello?

In the hospital room, my aunt *did* look exhausted. But she also looked beautiful, with her hair all messy and her skin glowing with sweat. "Hi, Meghan!" she said with a smile, and then . . . she was screaming bloody murder. A contraction had started, and my mother grabbed her little sister's hand and didn't let go. Nurses I hadn't even noticed surrounded the bed, and everyone seemed to forget I was there. I didn't want to leave, but I didn't know whether I could stay. Luckily, Lisa noticed I was still there, fear and excitement on my face.

"Meghan's still here?!" she shouted, and my mom looked up, surprised. I nodded to her, hoping she wouldn't send me back out into the waiting room.

"Meghan," Mom said, "you can stay. But you're going to need to mature real fast. You're going to see *everything*. Only stay in this room if you can handle that, promise?"

"I promise," I said, and I stepped up beside my aunt's bed to hold her other hand. I'm pretty sure that the rest of my friends spent their weekend watching TV, but I was a child doula helping my aunt give birth . . . and I was loving it. When the nurses told her it was time to push, Uncle Burton looked like he was about to pass out, so my mom and I each held one of Lisa's legs and counted down from ten, screaming "Pusssshhhhh!" when we hit one.

My mom wasn't lying; I saw *everything*. I saw a doctor put his fingers in my aunt's vagina when the contractions were getting closer together; I saw the crazy look in her eye when the doctor told her to push harder; I saw what came out of her when she started pushing . . . and it wasn't just a baby.

"You're doing great!" I screamed, even though I had no way of knowing if that was true. "Let's get this baby out of you!"

I saw the top of baby Marcus's head starting to emerge, and I couldn't believe what I was witnessing. Lisa's entire body was transforming and shifting and expanding to push out a brand-new person. She was amazing; this *experience* was amazing. And when Marcus finally squeezed out (I'm sorry, but it's really the only word for it), I felt . . . terrible. His face was squished, and he had a conehead. All that work, and my aunt had a little alien? Seeing my face and reading my mind, a nurse told me that this is what all babies look like at first, and soon my cousin would be cute. Marcus was already pressed against my aunt's bare chest, and she was crying into his head. A long, alien-like umbilical cord pressed between them, pulsating.

The doctor asked Lisa's husband if he wanted to cut the cord, but he shook his head, so the doctor *passed me the giant scissors.* I was so excited, I started imagining my future career as a nurse. Maybe other kids would have been freaked out, but I was honored and humbled by the entire experience, so much so that I showed up to do the same thing *on purpose* when Lisa had another baby a few years later. And even though I'd seen her do it before, it was me who cried when she delivered her next child.

I'm sure my parents were convinced I was destined to be a doula or a teen mom (no shade—that's one of the best reality shows of all time), but I was never in a hurry to be a mother; I just knew it was waiting for me, on the other side of some invisible door. I didn't know that it was possible to miss people you haven't met yet, but by my twenties I longed for my children. If you ever saw me in Target crying at the sight of diapers when I was just twenty-two, I'm sorry if I ruined your shopping trip. Personally, I thought I was crazy.

"Why am I crying about diapers when I don't even have a husband yet?" I asked my therapist, preparing to be told I was in the midst of losing my mind.

"Because you're already mothering your future children," she told me, with absolutely zero judgment.

Isn't that beautiful? I wasn't weird; I was *mothering*. This was already a part of my identity, and I didn't need to be ashamed of it just because I was young and only dreaming about my future. That acceptance meant that when I met my now-husband, Daryl, I wasn't afraid to tell him what I wanted: marriage, kids, and a family. I wrote a song called "Marry Me" one month into dating him and sang it to him in our hotel room while I was on tour. A tad aggressive, sure, but I walked down the aisle to that same song.

As I write this, I'm mothering a very real baby named Riley. He has my eyes and his dad's red hair, and he has both our hearts clenched in his little, powerful hands. (He's also pulled out a lot of my hair, but we'll get to that later.)

MEET TEAM MAMA

I'm a lot of things in the world, but I'm not a doctor, a registered dietitian, a personal trainer, or a doula. But because I have access to the best of the best—and because I love you so much, bestie—I pulled together the women who have been with me through every step of my own motherhood journey to bring their expertise to you.

REBECCA STANTON
@ @rebeccabroxfit

The first word that comes to mind with Rebecca is *badass*. I was *not* in the best shape of my life when I got pregnant, but Rebecca has helped me stay healthy through pregnancy, birth, and early motherhood. Rebecca spent years as a dancer in her hometown of Topeka, Kansas, before moving to Los Angeles and making the transition into personal training. With Rebecca, fitness is about far more than just looks: she encourages all her clients to "be inspired to inspire," to think about health more than appearances, and to appreciate our bodies for everything they do for us. Rebecca is certified by the National Academy of Sports Medicine and holds prenatal and postpartum certifications. She's guided several clients safely through pregnancy, encouraging them to love and nourish their bodies before, during, and after giving birth.

KRISTY MORRELL, RD

Don't let the *dietitian* title scare you; Kristy isn't the kind of person who makes you give up every food you love in the name of health. If she did, I wouldn't be working with her! Kristy worked as a sports dietitian for the University of Southern California and the Los Angeles Kings, educating athletes on proper nutrition to enhance performance, and is currently in private practice specializing in eating disorders, sports performance, weight management, and the impact of dietary habits. Kristy is a mama of two boys, and her passion is helping people change their relationship with food: no fads, no diets, no gimmicks. She believes in listening to *and* appreciating your body. See why I love her?

DR. KARYN SOLKY, OB-GYN

Dr. Solky is a graduate of the University of California, Berkeley, and the UCLA School of Medicine, and is an attending physician at Cedars-Sinai Medical Center here in LA. She's also a legend, the doctor's doctor, and the woman who showed me that there was hope. Dr. Solky was my *second* gyno and took me on as a patient halfway through my pregnancy. She raised the bar on the standard of care (which I didn't realize I deserved). She listened to every ridiculous question and answered kindly and thoroughly. She told me tough news so calmly—and with a smile—that I didn't even realize it wasn't the best news. From the first appointment, I felt like we'd been friends for years, and now . . . well, she's stuck with me forever.

DARYL SABARA

Yes, I married the kid from *Spy Kids*, and yes, he lives up to every lyric in "Dear Future Husband." I swear he's better than anything I could have ever dreamed of, and I dream *big*. He's perfect for me in every way, but he set the bar *high* for how a partner should show up in pregnancy— to the point where my friends have asked him to do a master class about it. He'll pop up in this book from time to time to give his perspective.

MAMA'S RULES

I know from experience that motherhood is a team sport. And every sport has rules, right? I'd like to set some for us right now. Raise your right hand and repeat after me (not for reals, but you can if you want):

1. Mamas don't judge one another. Unless you see a mother putting her baby in danger or breaking a law, let's cool it on the mom judgment. This experience is hard enough without wondering if our friends are gossiping about whether we're cloth diapering or using disposables. (TBH I did not have the time, energy, or interest in rinsing feces out of a piece of wet cotton, but I give a standing ovation to every parent who chooses this for their kid.)

2. Mamas don't judge themselves. This is the hardest rule and the most serious one. You're doing something you've never done before, and I *insist* you become your biggest fan.

3. Mama knows best. All the information out there can have your head swimming. Remember that you are the leading expert on yourself, even when you're doing something you've never done before. If something doesn't feel right to you, it probably isn't right. Believe in yourself. You got this.

4. Mama does her best (and has the right to change her mind). We do the best we can with what we know at the time, and every day we learn more about ourselves and our babies. It is normal and totally acceptable to change your mind about *anything* related to this journey (just check with your doctor first).

PART ONE

TRIMESTER ONE

ONE

LET'S GET PREGNANT

I spent the better part of my twenties wanting to have a family and also making sure I didn't get pregnant. I had a crazy career, I had a busy life, and, most importantly, I wanted to have kids with the right person, at the right time. Pregnancy seemed like an option that I could just turn on like preferences in an app. Who am I, Gen Z? Well, I *do* manifest like Gen Z. I'm the girl who wrote "Dear Future Husband" just to make sure that wherever he was, he knew my criteria for applying to be the Love of My Life. I've always known exactly what I wanted, and so did Daryl. But before he met me, he didn't think he'd ever get married, and he didn't even know if he wanted kids.

How I met Daryl is one of my favorite stories to tell, and it's even better when we tell it together because he'll pop in with details he thinks I forgot. (I didn't forget, babe. I was just moving the story along.) I was eighteen years old when we met, just a little baby songwriter invited to a party at a fancy house in the Hollywood Hills. I was visiting LA for work, feeling like the coolest person in the world, when the party got crashed. A bunch of guys walked in, and I heard people whispering that one of the guys was Juni from *Spy Kids*. Oh. My. God. I was immediately *starstruck,* y'all. So I did what my eighteen-year-old brain told me was the cool thing to do: I walked up to him and said, "Are you Spy Kids?" That's legit how I said it: "Are you Spy Kids?" Not "Are you Juni from *Spy Kids*?" He laughed, and he nodded, and when I went home that night, I replayed our cringey interaction and prayed he would forget it.

Daryl Says

Of course I hadn't forgotten! Meghan is unforgettable. And even though I used to hate when people did this, she was cute, so I really didn't mind.

Three years later, my career had blown up, and I was having the time of my life. But I'm a hopeless romantic, and I would stay up at night writing love songs and hoping like a Disney princess that true love would find me. My dad always told me, "If you stop obsessing over it, *that's* when love will find you." But that was impossible for me. I could never not think about it. I was on the hunt. I was twenty-one years old and acting like I'd been waiting for ages, but again, I am impatient, so I asked my friend Chloe Grace Moretz if she knew anyone who was cute and sweet, and she lit up. She told me that her best friend was the cutest, sweetest guy she'd ever met, that he was totally perfect. His name was Daryl, and he played Juni in *Spy Kids*.

Y'all. What are the chances?

She then set us up a double date with her and her boyfriend at the time, and then I prayed that in the three years that had passed since we last met, he'd forgotten that I was the girl who called him "Spy Kids."

He had not.

I Snapchatted him right before our date and asked him if he remembered, and when he typed back "Of course I remember," I was mortified. I thought he might cancel the date. Nope.

A few days later we were on our first date. Six days later we said "I love you," and five days after *that* I left on tour . . . and Daryl came with. From day one we were inseparable, and things just made sense. Just before we were set up on our first date, I'd written one of those hopelessly romantic songs of mine, called—wait for it—"Hopeless Romantic."

Bet we met at a party before
You were sweet and held open the door
Oh my, I should've said hi
So if you're out there
And hearing this song
Just know I'm here
And you're taking too long

I did not know when I wrote those lyrics that my future husband would be *a guy I met at a party before*! It was clearly meant to be, and Daryl felt the same way, which was surprising because he'd never seen himself as the marrying kind.

It was the second show date of the tour—day twelve of dating, to be exact—when he looked at me and said, "I never saw myself getting married or having kids . . . until I met you. I love you and I really see myself growing old with you."

I barked back at him, "You wanna marry me?!" I'm pretty sure I did the whole song and dance that Sandra Bullock does in *Miss Congeniality* when Benjamin Bratt falls in love with her (great movie, BTW). I was excited and cheesing, and then I sat down and wrote "Marry Me." Was this quick? Yep, but it made total sense to me: of course we loved each other, and of course we'd have a million babies. Or at least three to six babies. Daryl currently wants three or five, but I don't know about an uneven number.

Wanting kids is one of those things a lot of people wouldn't bring up in the early stages of dating, but those people aren't me. If Daryl hadn't brought it up that quickly, I would have. I feel like it's better to have your real wants and needs out in the open so you know early on whether this potential partner can meet them. If you don't want the same things in life, it's not the right person for you. It wouldn't have mattered how magical those first eleven days had been; if Daryl had looked me in the eye and told me he loved me but he didn't want kids? It would have been a deal breaker for me.

Now, people have a lot of opinions about when you should have kids. Have them too young and you're irresponsible. Wait too long and you're selfish. People love to let you know that the clock is ticking and time could run out.

Daryl and I got married on my twenty-fifth birthday. He was twenty-six years old, and people told us to wait a few years before having kids. A few years felt like a really long time, but my career was busy, and I was always working and traveling. Our life felt like a revolving door of hopping from a car to a plane to a new stage in a new city. I'm not complaining—I love my job. But in those chaotic days I didn't see how I could do it with a giant belly or swollen ankles, or how we'd lug around a baby stroller. Everyone who knew me knew that I wanted babies . . . ASAP. Knowing my mom had kids at twenty-four might have been a part of this, but I had to remind myself that she had a forty-three-year-old husband and their clock actually was ticking. My work supports a whole team of people, but to their credit they always told me that whenever I was ready to have kids, they'd be ready to support me.

And then, COVID-19 happened. There were no more shows and no more travel. Like a lot of people, we thought it would last a few weeks, maybe a few months. But when it became clear we weren't "going back to normal" any time soon, we took it as a sign that maybe it was time to try. If I had bad morning sickness or a complicated pregnancy, I wouldn't have to worry about traveling for work. We weren't going anywhere, so we wouldn't have to worry about paparazzi leaking the news. And besides, what else was there for two newlyweds to do once we'd watched everything on Netflix? We were home, we weren't going anywhere, and we'd made it a year and a half into our marriage. It was time to try. And time for my *obsession* to begin.

Doctor's Note

I'm Ready to Be a Mom. Now What?

I'm Dr. Solky, and I have the best job in the world. As an obstetrician-gynecologist (ob-gyn), I've spent my entire career caring for women through all stages of life. It's an honor to be a part of my patients' best and worst moments and to see them through so many life milestones. One of my favorite parts of my job is obstetrics—caring for pregnant women—and guiding my patients through the process of becoming mothers.

It's never too soon to talk to your provider; it gives us the chance to address any potential issues before they become urgent. Before conception, my patients and I go through their health history to make sure they're not on any medications that could be unsafe for a baby and that any underlying medical conditions that could affect their pregnancy are monitored and managed as well as possible. We also check their vaccinations; while you're pregnant, there are some vaccines you can't receive for diseases that you might have naturally lost immunity to over the years, so we'll want to make sure those are up-to-date. We'll also do a carrier screening for a panel of genetic disorders to make sure that mom isn't a carrier. If she is, we'll screen the partner. It sounds scary, but it's always best to make informed decisions about your family planning and to be able to address any issues before they become urgent.

I don't know what kind of an education you all got in high school, but I was told that penis plus vagina equals baby. Until the day I saw my cousin's gremlin face emerging from my aunt's vag, I hadn't really thought about how any of it . . . happened. When you're young, pregnancy seems like a thing that just *happens*. The internet is filled with advice on how to get pregnant: you can find entire diet plans, yoga moves, superstitions, spells, prayers, medical procedures, conspiracy theories, tests . . . it's easy to get overwhelmed. That's exactly what I did: I spent literal days watching YouTube and TikTok and Instagram videos of pregnant women telling the world what they did to get knocked up.

No, really, *every day* I searched "how to get pregnant" on YouTube and did whatever these random women told me to do. I was willing to try anything and made getting pregnant our job. Look, we do the best we can in the moment, but if I *could* go back in time? I'd tell myself to *chill*. We were having sex three times a day. Wake up: sex. A small break from work: sex. After dinner: sex. I love my husband and we had some good times, but I wasn't being very romantic. Let me tell you, nothing takes the sexiness out of sex like giving it a mission and making it an item on your to-do list.

Wait, there's one more thing that probably doesn't help: putting a menstrual cup inside yourself after sex to keep the sperm in longer. Yeah, I did that. I did that because a YouTuber said it "may" have worked for her . . . sad. Disclaimer: I am not suggesting you take medical advice from a YouTuber! But anyone who knows me knows I'm the most impatient person ever. So I was willing to try *anything*.

Daryl Says

Look, I love my wife very much and had *no* problem "trying" three times a day. What most people don't know is that when Meghan wants to achieve something, she obsesses over it until it happens.

She's not just "impatient"—she's the most impatient person I've ever met. That's an incredible quality . . . most of the time. It's part of what has made her so successful, and it's definitely one of the millions of reasons why I love her so much. She's a boss. But did I want a boss to tell me it was time to "perform" in the middle of a workday because she saw a YouTube video that told her to try a different position? Not really.

Meanwhile, it felt like I was watching everyone in the world *except* me get pregnant. Every announcement brought me happiness for the couple and frustration for me and my husband. All this research meant that I was slowly becoming a scientist with a degree from the University of Google. I knew in my head that pregnancy meant a series of biological dominoes all had to fall into place: the egg releasing, the right sperm breaking out from the pack, the fertilized egg implanting into your uterus and not getting stuck in a fallopian tube or just drifting out in your next period. When you think about it—*really* think about it—it's amazing that any of us are here at all, that all those microscopic events happened at the right time and right place . . . and made a person. Everyone on this Earth—even the really annoying people you can't stand—is a damn miracle. But in my heart I just thought, *Okay, so where is our miracle?* I popped my prenatal vitamins and spent thirty minutes after sex lying on my back with my legs up the wall while playing my Nintendo and hoping for the best.

I knew that it could take time to get pregnant, but as I've said, I have a patience problem, and I was freaking out after just two months of negative pregnancy tests. I know, I know, *chill.* But have you ever tried telling a woman who wants to be pregnant to *chill*? I wouldn't recommend it, especially after she gets her period. I swear, the period goes from being a minor inconvenience to the biggest "fuck you."

So I was in a mood; I was impatient. Where did I go? Back to

YouTube for more "tips on getting pregnant." A few clicks in, I found myself watching a segment from a TV show about getting pregnant. I was ready to hear some tips . . . and not ready to hear about how we were doing it wrong. The show suggested that we were having *too much sex* and not giving Daryl's body time to make more sperm. This, it turns out, might not actually be scientifically proven,[1] but either way, I didn't appreciate a scientist telling me that we were doing it wrong. Not sex itself—we're good at that—but we weren't having *fun*. We were stressed out and acting like it was a job, when really, we were taking the very first steps toward building a family.

Here's what I needed to focus on: *my body*. When it came down to it, pregnancy is just science. Crazy science. Listen: A tiny, microscopic egg is released from the fallopian tube and the clock starts ticking. It has twelve to twenty-four hours to be fertilized. To fertilize the egg, sperm have to go on a vicious *journey*, and of all the millions that should be in a single shot of sperm, just *one* is all it takes. I don't know how you'd even try to write out a math equation for your chances of getting pregnant, but that's crazy, right? Then I read that while your eggs just have that little window, sperm *can* live inside you for up to five days after sex *in the right conditions*.[2] What are those conditions? Don't ask me, because when I first heard that, I wasn't taking any chances. The way I acted, the window was always open and baby-making was a full-time job.

But not anymore: I ordered a box of ovulation testers and told Daryl we had a new plan: no sex. He was . . . confused. How would we make a baby without sex? Well, we'd *have* sex . . . in fourteen days, when and if I ovulated. He was sweet—he's always so sweet—and nodded along while I told him that every morning I would pee on one of these tests and wait for a smiley face to tell me I was ovulating. No smiley face? No sex. Was he super pumped about this new plan? No, not really, but he was a brave guy, and he survived.

And the morning I saw that smiley face, I jumped back in bed with Daryl and made it count.

Daryl Says

Okay, this is when I really wanted to block her access to YouTube. But here's what future dads need to know: your wife/girlfriend/ partner is going through a *lot* right now. It might not all be rational, but it's very emotional, and your job here is to be supportive, be a good listener . . . and yeah, wait two little weeks for sex if that's what she wants. She's carrying your baby for *nine months*! You can do two weeks. I recommend meditation, breath work, and as many distractions as possible.

AND NOW . . . WE WAIT

There's an excruciating part of getting pregnant you need to know about: the Two-Week Wait. Not the two weeks I made Daryl wait to have sex, but—you guessed it—the two weeks between ovulation and implantation, fourteen days for you to wonder whether a sperm found an egg and whether that fertilized egg has found a place in your uterus. The only way to tell it worked is for your body to build up enough of the pregnancy hormone beta-hCG that it can be detected in blood or pee. And while you're waiting . . . you just get to obsess over it.

My mom thought I was crazy counting down the days and obsessing over every little twinge that could have been implantation, but my YouTube besties? They got me. I spent the full two weeks watching YouTube videos to try to figure out what I was supposed to be feeling. Calm, beautiful women would look into the camera and whisper-talk, like, "Girl, if you're waiting . . . listen to your body." I tried! I spent the two-week wait feeling like everything my body did was a sign, but not a sign that I could read. Was that implantation I felt in my belly, or just a fart coming? Were my breasts tender because I was pregnant or because I was about to have my period? What about not feeling anything at all? Was that bad, or *was even that a symptom*?

IS IT PREGNANCY OR YOUR PERIOD?

Sore boobs

Cramps

Fatigue

Feeling emotional

Bloating

Light spotting

Trick question. It could be either! What a hilarious nightmare!

My boobs felt like . . . boobs. My body felt like . . . a body. The only difference this month was that I had zero symptoms (which convinced me that I was *definitely* not pregnant this time).

The morning that marked two weeks, I tried to play it cool and distract myself. We woke up and went on a hike to celebrate my friend Tommy's birthday. It's one of our favorite hikes, with a gradual incline and a winding path that tricks you into thinking you're just on a walk—until you see all of Los Angeles spread out below you. We were in the thick of the pandemic, so this was the best birthday celebration we could come up with, and I was excited to finally get out of the house. But from the minute we stepped on the trail, I was *winded*. I'm always winded while going up steep hills or any staircase, but this was different. I was dangling off my husband, trying to fight gravity. I felt like crap, and I *knew* I was about to get my period. I didn't have any pregnancy symptoms, and I'd have to tell Daryl *again* that it hadn't worked.

When we got home, I was hot and sweaty and definitely in a mood. I was certain I started my period on this brutal hike. But when I got home and went to the bathroom, I saw no blood. I decided I *had* to take a pregnancy test before my shower. You know, just to prove to myself I wasn't pregnant. Mind you, I wasn't days late. I wasn't even *hours* late. If I really thought I was pregnant, I would've filmed this moment and would've waited till I wasn't a hot, sweaty mess.

"I don't know why I'm doing this," I said to Daryl while I was peeing on the stick. "I don't have any symptoms. It's just going to say *not pregnant* and then I'll be depressed and cramping all day."

I stepped into the shower to turn it on and feel sorry for myself, feeling the water heat up as it ran over my hands. Meanwhile, Daryl was staring at the test I'd left on the counter. When I turned, he had the biggest smile I'd ever seen. This is the moment I'll remember forever, because it's so perfectly us: Daryl said, "You're *pregnant!*" And without missing a beat, I shouted, "*No fucking way!*" I was laughing, and I was crumpling, sweaty and naked and collapsing into my husband's arms while we cried tears of joy.

Daryl Says

After all her hard work, it felt unfair that I saw it first. But it's one of the best moments of my life, and I'll cherish it forever. Third time's the charm!

TWO

PRE-PREGNANCY CHECKLIST

I love to be prepared, even if it means derailing a meeting so I can make sure everyone on the team knows the newest "fun fact" about pregnancy that is really only fun to me. We started trying during the COVID-19 pandemic, when everything was scary and uncertain. Looking at the news or Twitter was like being hit with a fire hose of stress and fear, and I was lucky enough to be physically safe and still have work, even if I was stuck at home. All the research I was doing on pregnancy is a part of my personality for sure, but it was also a way to calm my anxious brain: the more information I have, the more control I feel over a situation, even when a situation is totally out of my control.

I am always the first person to a meeting, I deep-dive down rabbit holes whenever I'm interested in something, and I *love* a to-do list. The following list is not the be-all and end-all, and there is a lot on this list that I didn't think about until after the fact, or didn't *need* to think about . . . but you might. Every family and situation is unique, so use this as a jumping-off point while you plan for your future as a family.

TALK TO YOUR PARTNER

I mean, duh. But there's a lot to talk about once you've both agreed that you want to have kids. When do you want to officially try? What is your plan in the event of infertility? Are you open to medical assistance to help you conceive? Nobody wants to think about that last one, but having the conversation before you need to is going to make a potentially devastating situation at least a *bit* easier.

INTERVIEW YOUR FAMILY

Okay, this sounds serious, but ask your parents about any family history with pregnancy loss or birth defects. These are questions your provider will ask you, too, so it's good to be prepared.

EVALUATE YOUR BUDGET

Everyone tells you babies are expensive, but pregnancy can be too. Even if you have great insurance, you're going to have out-of-pocket expenses. Those co-pays can add up! So can maternity clothes, vitamins, childcare costs, and all the gear you'll eventually need for this new baby (more on that in the third trimester). Even if you plan your budget down to the penny, things always come up. Some might be little, but the thing about complications is that they're unexpected. A friend of mine is a waitress whose morning sickness was really just all-the-time sickness, and she ended up needing to have four teeth pulled unexpectedly as a result. That's not cheap and nothing she could have planned for. Another friend of mine started putting away the average weekly day care cost in her city *right when she got pregnant.* By the time the baby arrived, they had almost a year's worth of day care costs covered. I'm not saying you have to go *that* crazy, but having a handle on your monthly income and expenses before you throw a baby into the works is *crucial*.

CHECK YOUR LEAVE POLICY AT WORK

America is *way* behind the rest of the world on parental leave. While our Canadian friends get a full year off to care for a new child, Americans are considered lucky if they're eligible for the Family and Medical Leave Act, which gives *eligible employees* twelve weeks of parental leave (unpaid).[1] Another option is to take six weeks of short-term disability at about 60 percent pay.[2]

It's bad, and we gotta change it, but in the meantime, you need to make sure you're fully aware of what your employer does—and does not—provide. Some smaller employers may not have parental coverage at all.

Check your benefits paperwork to make sure your plan covers maternity care and to find out the details of any parental leave policy. If this isn't clearly spelled out in writing somewhere, reach out to your HR person (or your boss) and ask: What benefits do we provide for pregnant women in this company?

Mamas, this is important: your employer cannot use a pregnancy (or your desire to get pregnant) as a reason to fire you, deny you a promotion, or affect your job in any way.[3] I was nervous to tell my team about my pregnancy, and I'm the boss! I can only imagine how nerve-racking it would be if you aren't in a supportive environment, so remember that you do have rights. Your employer can't ask if you're pregnant, if you're trying to get pregnant, or anything like that. Your body, your business!

CALL YOUR INSURANCE

As I said, having a baby isn't cheap, even without medical complications. Ask your insurance provider:

- What appointments are covered? At what percentage?
- What is my out-of-pocket maximum?
- What providers are in-network?
- What kind of coverage do I have if there are complications?
- Does the plan cover childbirth classes? A breast pump?
- What are my deductible and co-pay amounts for maternal care?
- Are my doctor and birth facility covered by the plan?
- Post-delivery, how long am I covered for a hospital stay?
- In the event of birth complications, how does that coverage change?
- When and how do I add my baby to the health plan?
- Does the plan cover certified nurse midwives and nonhospital birth centers or a home birth? (It's a hard pass for me, but shout-out to all my home-birthing mama friends!)

LEARN YOUR CYCLE

I was a late bloomer here, so learn from me: learn about your body. I've heard a lot of moms rave about *Taking Charge of Your Fertility* by Toni Weschler, but I used apps (and there are a lot of them). Before you sign up to share your cycle and pregnancy data with any app, review the privacy policies to confirm that they don't share your personal data with any third parties and that you understand what you're signing up for. However you learn it, knowing how regular your cycle is, when you're ovulating, and the best times for you to "try" is crucial.

TAKE PRENATAL SUPPLEMENTS

Your body needs iron to support a fetus and a placenta and folic acid to help your baby's brain and spinal cord develop. I started taking supplements months before I even tried to get pregnant because they do amazing things for your hair and your nails. Plus, they come in gummy form now (*yum*), so you don't have to swallow a pill.

Keep It Moving with Rebecca ————————————

Women are hard on ourselves (shocking, I know!), especially when trying to conceive. We want to get everything right, and I get that. Now's the time to start building endurance and strength for the physically demanding road ahead. I suggest a yoga class (not hot yoga!) to help relax your mind and strengthen your body. And I know nobody wants to hear this, but stressing out will not help you get pregnant, so if you can already feel your stress level rising, it's time to try some meditation or gentle movement (a walk is great!).

GO TO THE DENTIST

Apparently, all these changes affect your *whole* body, including your teeth and gums?! Keep those choppers healthy, mama.

CALL THE MIDWIFE. OR THE OB . . . OR THE DOULA . . . OR DON'T. NO PRESSURE, SERIOUSLY.

Choosing your care team for your pregnancy is very personal. Like, *very* personal. These people are going to be seeing parts of you that you haven't even seen, and ensuring you're in the right set of hands is crucial to feeling safe and supported during your pregnancy. I went with an obstetrician (OB), but I have mama friends who swear by their doula or their midwife. There are entire *books* dedicated to these professions, but I thought a li'l cheat sheet might be helpful while you're in the planning stages.

	Who They Are	What They Do	Their Qualifications	When to Call Them
Ob-gyn	An obstetrician-gynecologist is a medical doctor who specializes in women's reproductive health.	An ob-gyn cares for your health during the pregnancy and also delivers the baby. They're the doctor you see for your yearly gynecological visit, which I hope you never skip (though yes . . . I have).	They've been alllll the way through medical school and three to seven years in internships and residencies.	Well, hopefully you already have. But schedule an appointment when you're ready to try to get pregnant to talk about any preexisting conditions, your current medications, and any concerns you might have. Did I do this? Nope! I just dove right in.
Midwife	This sounds very old-timey, but certified nurse midwives are modern medical professionals who specialize in women's health care.[4]	Depending on the state, they provide care from gynecological exams to family planning to labor and delivery (but not C-sections). They aren't doctors, but many of them practice under a doctor's supervision or consult with an ob-gyn.	Certified nurse midwives have graduated from a certified nurse midwifery program and have passed a national exam.	Midwives typically serve women who are low-risk and want fewer medical interventions, or options like a home or water birth. You can see a midwife for a pre-pregnancy check-in or meet with one once you're knocked up.

Doula (sometimes called a *birth coach*)	If you're a crunchy mama who wants to avoid being induced and do it all naturally . . . man, good for you. Your doula is your coach, your advocate, and a teammate for you *and* your partner.	A doula is your personal guide for the emotional *and* physical parts of the pregnancy journey and beyond. Many of them also provide hands-on follow-up care when you and baby get home. Lots of people use a doula even with an ob-gyn or a midwife, as an extra support person and advocate during the birth process.	A doula is not usually a medical professional, but they should be certified through an organization like DONA International.	Interview doulas when you're pregnant. You can find certified doulas at DONA.org or through word of mouth (from people you trust, not randoms!).

If you're feeling overwhelmed, take a breath. Then take another. Now smile and say, "Wow, I'm stunning." You don't have to have it all figured out right now, or even before the baby comes. Also, whenever I thought I was unprepared or doing things wrong, I'd remember that our eighty-year-old family friend was told *by her doctor* to smoke when she was pregnant to "keep her weight down" and "have small babies." At least we aren't doing that, right? For real, though, you can't be smoking or vaping or drinking alcohol or anything once you're pregnant; it's not the 1950s anymore and that shit's bad for your baby.

THREE

I'M PREGNANT (I THINK)

Here's something that makes zero sense: your first trimester of pregnancy starts the first day of your *last* period. About five minutes after Daryl told me I was pregnant, I was back on my phone, downloading every single pregnancy app available on an iPhone. For real, every pregnancy app was on my phone, and I refreshed them all religiously, as though there would be breaking news on what was happening in my uterus . . . from an app downloaded by literally millions of people. I even downloaded them all on Daryl's phone too. I opened those apps all day long as if new information would magically pop up. But I did learn some things, like that I couldn't have sushi anymore (bummer) and that I was somehow already two weeks pregnant even though the test was still wet.

I also learned my due date: February 14. We didn't plan it, but yeah, we made a Valentine's Day love child and yes, it went straight to my head. I told everyone, "It's because Daryl and I are soulmates," and left out the fact that I'd also learned that a "due date" is really just a guesstimate and not the day your baby will actually pop into the world.

I called my doctor right away, because obviously I needed to get in there—I was pregnant! But here's the thing: your first appointment is usually about eight weeks after your last period. I had six weeks to go (or so they said—you know I pushed for an earlier appointment), and I wanted all the information I could find, and fast. What was I going to feel? What was happening? And most importantly, was I actually pregnant? I didn't *feel* pregnant! Also, I was *dying* to know whether there was a tiny little blonde diva floating inside me or an itty-bitty Spy Kid. I typed in the date of my last period and was told our baby was . . . a poppy seed? Really? A microscopic poppy seed? I scrolled forward to find out that in a week, our baby would be the size of a sesame seed. It would take weeks, apparently, for this baby to grow to the size of a pea. I wouldn't know the sex until a blood test at ten weeks! I get that it's not an overnight process, but my impatient ass was freaking out.

Every day those first few weeks, I'd wake up and look at my belly. It looked like . . . my belly. Like a normal, everyday belly. What. The. Hell?

"Do I look pregnant?" I'd ask Daryl, and he'd smile and nod.

"Hell yeah you look pregnant, babe!"

"Seriously, though, is there even a baby in there? Like for real?"

He didn't get it. I wanted to look pregnant-pregnant. I wanted to have a big, round belly that announced to every stranger on the street that there was a *baby* in here, even if we weren't really seeing any strangers anywhere because of COVID. But trust that if I passed someone on the hiking trail or had food delivered, I would tell them "I'm pregnant!" like it was the most normal thing in the world to tell a stranger who is dropping off burritos for dinner. The pregnancy was just ours, which is beautiful in a lot of ways, but also really lonely. Because one of the thrills I imagined of being pregnant for the first time was sharing the experience with other mamas-to-be. But *none* of my friends were even close to being pregnant. They all watched me in awe, like, "We are so glad you are doing this before us so we can learn from you." There are groups where women who are all due around the same time meet regularly, and I wanted that! I wanted a little group of friends who could all talk about our experiences and our symptoms. Even though—and this was weird to me—I wasn't really having any symptoms.

TYPICAL FIRST-TRIMESTER SYMPTOMS[1]

Weird cravings . . . or sudden icks

Darkened areolas

Mood swings (blame the hormones)

Headaches

Lower back pain

Nausea

Fatigue

Light spotting (not cool!)

Constipation (again, blame the hormones)

Peeing more (weird, right?)

MY FIRST-TRIMESTER SYMPTOMS

Being sleepy

End of list. That's literally all I experienced . . . sorry!

My boobs felt normal. My body felt normal. I was pooping like normal. The only big sign I felt in these weeks was *exhaustion*. I'm not a big napper, but in that first trimester, I could curl up nearly anywhere and fall into a deep, beautiful sleep.

My first OB appointment was strange. COVID meant that I went to the appointment without Daryl (the policy was mamas only, or I'd have rolled up with Daryl, my mom, possibly my brothers, Ryan and Justin, and my entire team). It also meant masking up and staying six feet apart from everyone in the waiting room (kinda weird that we used to just cuddle up next to strangers, but also weird to avoid one another this aggressively).

My doctor also didn't make me feel great. I know it's not a doctor's job to be your friend, but I felt like I was bugging him. Even in a huge COVID spike and without any partners or guests allowed, this place was *busy*. The first appointment means a lot of paperwork, and I felt so unprepared and naive when I sat down to fill it out alone, without my husband or my mom. It took me so long the doctor made a joke: "What are you writing, your autobiography?" I was mortified. *If I can't even fill out these forms, how am I gonna have a baby and keep them alive?*

The earliest weeks of pregnancy felt like walking on eggshells: one in four pregnancies end in miscarriage,[2] and that statistic terrified me. If it took a perfect series of events to even get pregnant, how fragile was the process of staying pregnant? I wanted to wrap myself in a cocoon to keep me and the baby safe, but I was also working on a Christmas album and I had a music video to shoot . . . during the pandemic. Could I dance without shaking the baby loose? If I gained weight, would my ankles break if I wore heels?

These might seem like silly questions, but this was the biggest, most important experience of my life so far and the doctor acted like I was the stupidest person he'd ever encountered. "You're twenty-six and healthy," he snipped. "You're not going to miscarry."

At this point, I pulled out my antidepressant, which at the time was 5 mg of lorazepam and 30 mg of citalopram. I told him, "My psychiatrist said it was okay to be on the citalopram, but I should stop the lorazepam."

He quickly waved his hand and said, "Oh, you can throw those candies away."

I was shattered. I felt shame, anger, and disappointment all at the same time. But I was also too submissive to say how I felt, so I didn't say anything. I just thought to myself, *I need a new OB.*

Then he did a quick vaginal exam. I felt awkward and was still pretty nervous, so I asked him "Does it look pregnant?" while he was investigating me. I was only kind of joking, but the way he laughed didn't feel like he was in on the joke; it felt like he was laughing at me. Maybe it's because he said, "You're like one hour pregnant; relax." I didn't relax; I just forced myself to giggle, shoved down my uncomfortable feelings, and counted the seconds until we were done.

Overall, the appointment felt rushed. I didn't feel heard, and I didn't feel any safer, I just felt . . . stupid and silly. Major red flag, friends. *Major.*

PRENATAL APPOINTMENT SCHEDULE

This depends on your pregnancy risks and the tests you opt into, but a standard schedule is:

4–28 weeks	Every four weeks
28–36 weeks	Every two weeks
36–40 weeks	Every week!

YOUR FIRST APPOINTMENT

It goes without saying, but I sure wish someone had said this to me: Your provider should not make you feel stupid, or silly, or unwelcome. You deserve to be treated with respect and to feel seen and heard through this process.

This first appointment *should* be long: they should ask a million questions about you and your family health history, take your blood, and run a bunch of tests. But your appointment is yours, so make sure you ask your questions too! No question is a stupid question, especially if you've never done this before. Make a list on your phone if you have to. I did that for every single appointment until birth, and it was so beyond helpful. Some questions to get you started:

- What screenings do you recommend for me based on my family's medical history?
- Do you see any reason for me to modify my current fitness routine or any of my other habits?
- Who do I call if I'm concerned about something? Do you have a nurse line?
- Is this weird pain normal?
- What's your approach to labor and delivery? (If you know you want a home birth, or a hospital birth that includes a birth coach or a doula, this is the time to make sure your provider is on board with your preferences.)
- Are there any additional screenings or tests you'd recommend based on my medical history? (This shit can get expensive, so ask in advance so you have time to research the cost and check with your insurance before you do anything.)

I was nervous about losing the pregnancy, but we also had work to do, so I shot the music video for "Make You Dance" at my house because I was too afraid to go anywhere with the pandemic going on. I was sweaty, my boobs looked *huge*, and I didn't want to show my body even though *literally nobody could tell I was pregnant with a poppy seed*. The director let me put on flowy dresses and kept the camera right on my face. Every time I sang "Got my rosé, been drinking since one . . ." I broke into an involuntary smile. I was *not* drinking rosé; I had a big, beautiful secret growing inside of me.

But did I *feel* beautiful? Honestly . . . no. I'm five foot five and I've always been thick by Hollywood standards, but when I got pregnant with Riley, I was at my heaviest weight I've ever been at 185 pounds, and I just didn't feel good about myself. And even though I know this should have been the furthest thought from my mind, I was worried about my weight and about the weight I would gain as the pregnancy progressed. Would that be healthy for me? For the baby? And yeah, I have done a lot of work on my own body positivity, but we still live in a culture that celebrates being skinny, and I've never fit that mold.

What I'm trying to say is this: body-image stuff is hard, and getting pregnant is not a magic cure for this. Guys, I hate this! I don't want us worrying about our weight and our appearance while our bodies are doing the actual *miracle* of making a person. But I'm not gonna lie to you, either: I did not feel great about my body before I got pregnant, and I didn't feel great about my body when I *got* pregnant. I didn't *want* to gain any more weight; I just wanted my belly to inflate like a big balloon so I could wear all the cute maternity clothes instead of men's XXL pajama pants and hoodies. I also really wanted to be healthy, but I was *terrified* that if I worked out, I would hurt the baby. Seriously y'all, I would go on the treadmill *gripping* my belly as though a little stroll was going to be too much for my uterus. The internet is filled with hot pregnant ladies running marathons and lifting weights and doing all kinds of crazy shit, but I know everyone is different and I didn't know what was and wasn't okay for *my* body.

And this brought me to two of the most transformational relation-ships for the way I feel about my body: my relationship with my trainer, Rebecca, and my dietitian, Kristy. I didn't get to work with them until my second trimester, but their approach to fitness and food helped shift my thinking and my entire pregnancy experience, which is why I had to make sure to bring their wisdom to you too.

FOUR

FIRST-TRIMESTER FOOD AND FITNESS

Keep It Moving with Rebecca

Let's start with the ground rules. Okay, maybe *rules* is a little strong. These are more like guidelines from a person who has dedicated years of her life to helping her clients feel their best before, during, and after pregnancy. You notice what I said there, right? I said *feel* their best. Because fitness is about more than looks, and when it comes to pregnancy, it's not at *all* about how you look.

I had a client who told me in her first trimester, "I don't want to get fat." I wasn't surprised to hear that at all. We live in a culture where fat is "bad," and we're constantly told that our looks are the most important thing; that mentality doesn't just turn off when you get pregnant. We know that the most important thing is a healthy baby, but we also know that Western culture loves for women to be thin and in shape. But I do think that we can do our best individually to shift that culture, so I gave this client an affirmation to say aloud for the rest of her pregnancy:

I want to gain weight if that's the best thing for my baby.

Do you know how hard that was for her to say? It might be hard for you to say too. It might be hard for you to believe. But pregnant bodies are truly miraculous, and in the months to come your body is going to do its best to create a healthy baby. So if and when you struggle with your body image, I have another affirmation for you. You can write it on your mirror in dry-erase marker, say it aloud, or put it on a sticky note where you'll see it every day:

It's not about how I look. It's about what my baby needs.

●

Once you've talked with your doctor and understand any pre-existing conditions or personal limitations, the rules of prenatal fitness are simple:

Pay attention to how you feel. Tired is fine—you *will* be tired from growing a whole person inside you!—but no workout should feel painful. If it hurts, stop. Just stop. No trainer or app or YouTube video should push you to the point of pain. When your body says rest, you rest, even if the circuit you're following calls for more reps. You're not exercising to win an award; you're exercising to build strength and endurance for childbirth and beyond.

Nothing new (for now). With the exception of walking or gentle yoga, pregnancy is not the time to add a new fitness endeavor to your life. If you're already a runner, great! But if you're not, this is not the time to sign up for a marathon. If you're already a powerlifter, that's awesome! But this is not the time to sign up for CrossFit. Stick with what you know, and follow the first rule!

Modify as needed. When you can't run, you walk. When you need to walk slower, you slow down. When you need to stop, you stop.

Physical activity should never be a punishment: your body is a gift and your ability to move is a blessing. So above all else, I hope you treat yourself with kindness and respect during your pregnancy—and for every day afterward.

First-Trimester Exercises

Aside from low-impact activities like swimming (I truly love swimming—get in a pool if you can!), walking, and yoga (again, not heated), these are two of my favorite circuits to do with my pregnant clients. Follow the "rules" and pay attention to how you feel—and keep that core engaged! You're going to need a lot of core strength to get through pregnancy and childbirth. Imagine zipping your abdomen together like you zip a winter coat: that's how an engaged core should feel. There are 2 sets here. Aim for 8 to 10 reps of each exercise, cycling through the set three times (unless your body tells you otherwise!).

Equipment Needed:

Dumbbells (5-to-8-pound weights or whatever you feel comfortable with)
Exercise mat (a rug or carpet works fine too)

Your Affirmation:

It's not about how I look. It's about what my baby needs.

SET 1

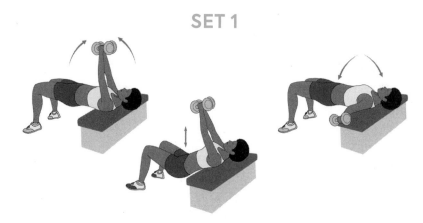

Hip-Thrust Dumbbell Chest Fly

Each rep of this exercise includes two motions: the hip thrust *and* the chest fly.

First, lie face up with your upper back on a bench and feet flat on the ground. Push the dumbbells above your face, parallel with each other like an 11. Drop your hips to the ground and lift them back up. When your hips are back up, pull the weights apart, lowering them in line with your shoulders, and then raise them back up to the starting position to prepare for another hip thrust. Imagine with every chest fly that your hands are tracing up and down a rainbow with the weights.

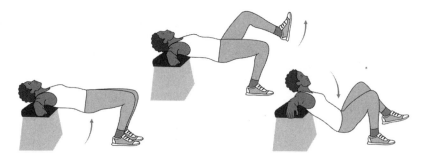

Single-Leg Hip Thrust

Lie face up with your upper back on a bench and feet flat on the ground. Lift one leg off the ground and bring that bent knee toward your chest. While holding this position, lower your hips toward the ground and back up again to the starting position. Repeat for additional reps, doing an equal number of reps on both sides.

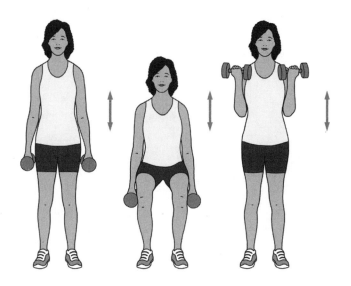

Deadlift Curl

Here's another two-parter, this one combining a deadlift and a bicep curl. Stand upright with your legs shoulder-width apart and dumbbells at your sides. With a straight back, hinge at the hips and bend your knees until you feel your glutes activate. Keep your knees at a soft bend; this is not a squat! Pushing from your heels, stand back up to your starting position and bend your arms at the elbows, bringing them toward your shoulders.

SET 2

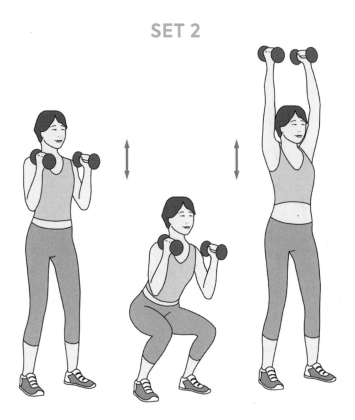

Dumbbell Squat to Press

Squats are amazing . . . when you do them right. Start in a standing position with your dumbbells at your shoulders, palms facing each other. Squat by bending your knees and sitting back with your hips, as if you were going to sit in an invisible chair. Pushing through your heels, stand back up as you press the dumbbells overhead, arms straight and elbows at your ears. Bring the dumbbells back to starting position and repeat movement for additional reps.

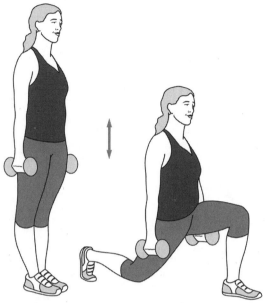

Alternating Reverse Lunge

Start in a standing position, holding the dumbbells at your sides. Step one leg back and bend both knees until they are both at a 90-degree angle, then step back in, bringing your feet back together. Repeat on the opposite side by stepping back with the other leg.

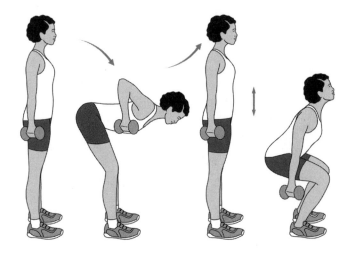

Bent-Over Row to Sumo Squat

Start with your feet a little wider than shoulder-width apart—this is the "sumo" part of the exercise—and your toes slightly turned out, weights in your hands.

Hinge forward so your back is parallel with the ground, and pull the weights up to your rib cage, bending your elbows to a 90-degree angle.

Lower your weights and stand up.

Keep your sumo stance and move into a sumo squat position, sitting back into that invisible chair with this wider stance and lowering your body toward the ground.

Stand up and start over.

Let's Eat with Kristy

Food is about more than just nutrition. Food is a source of comfort and connection, and for a lot of us, it has deep emotional and psychological roots. Some of us were raised in the Clean Plate Club or told "Take all you like, but eat all you take." Some of us have been on diets since before we could spell the word or grew up without access to good nutrition or regular meals. It's a *lot*, and when you add in that you're now responsible for the life that is growing inside you . . . well, that's a lot too. So we're going to start with a mantra not just for pregnancy but for every day:

I'm doing the best I can.

You are, and you always have been, even on the days you didn't think so. The first trimester especially, a lot of women find even their favorite foods unappealing. It's fine if you can't eat anything green for the first few weeks of pregnancy; just remember to take your prenatal vitamin and to get as much variety in your diet as possible. You don't need to shop at only the most expensive, organic grocery stores to eat well, and you don't need to judge yourself for not having Pinterest-level meals every single day. No fresh produce at your local store? Frozen is fine! Starving in an airport where the only option is fast food? Make the best choice you can!

Often, the conversation around nutrition is about restriction and punishment, but not here. I want the conversation in this book and everywhere to shift to a mindset of love and appreciation for who we are and what we have. With every bite or sip from this moment on, your goal is to love yourself and this baby, who is absorbing everything you consume. Because once this baby is out in the world, they're *still* absorbing: whether you realize it or not, they soak up messages about food and wellness the same way you did when you were little. We have an awesome responsibility and opportunity as mothers to make sure they absorb healthy, loving messages about their bodies . . . and to work on reprogramming our own messaging too.

KRISTY'S "RULES"

Having a loving relationship with ourselves and nutrition does require us to change some of our deeply ingrained habits, so I give these rules to all my clients.

No eating from the box. Or the jar, the bag, the container it came in. Even if you're just grabbing a handful of chips, take the time to put them in a bowl.

Read the ingredients. Get into the habit of reading the packaging and knowing what's in your food. In the nineties, when dietary fat was considered "bad," packaged food became packed with sugar. Now that "sugar-free" is a selling point, there are countless other additives on the ingredient list.

Hydrate. Water is essential for cellular function and for moving nutrients through your body. Aim for two to three liters of water a day. Meghan went up to a gallon a day while pregnant with Riley and never stopped!

Appreciate your food. Before you take a bite, take a moment to show gratitude for the food you have and the meal or snack you're about to enjoy.

Slow down. Sometimes we're busy, I know, but meals should take fifteen to twenty minutes to eat. That's not that long, but when you're used to slamming back a meal while sitting at your desk, it can feel like an eternity. Take your time! Set down your fork, lean back in your chair, talk to the people at the table with you. Did I say *table*? Yeah . . .

No more couch meals. Or computer meals. Or—if you can help it—meals behind the wheel. I know we're all busy, but eating your meal at a dining table is a way to treat your meal times as special and sacred and to help you slow down and enjoy them.

Be your own mom. You know how the best moms always had snacks and water ready for their kids? Well, from this moment on, you do not leave your house without a snack and some water!

FIRST-TRIMESTER FOODS

In every trimester, there are nutrients and foods that are important for the development of your growing baby. Think of these as guidelines, and remember that you need to be realistic with yourself based on how you feel, what's available to you, and the pregnancy symptoms you're experiencing. Be gentle with yourself and show yourself compassion. You do not need to stress out about eating "perfectly." *You are doing the best you can.*

The American Pregnancy Association recommends avoiding deli meats, fish that are typically high in mercury, smoked seafood, raw eggs or meat, unpasteurized milk, alcohol, and some soft cheeses.[1] Guidelines are always changing, so check with your health-care provider about the foods you should be eating and avoiding.

What It Is	What It Does	Where to Get It
Omega-3 fatty acids	Critical for brain and tissue development in utero	Chia seeds, salmon, mackerel, and walnuts
DHA	Critical for brain and tissue development in utero	Cold-water fish like mackerel and salmon
Healthy fats	Critical for brain and tissue development in utero	Nuts and nut butters, seeds, whole-milk dairy, and avocado
Folate	Helps with the development of the baby's nervous system (brain and spinal cord)	Leafy greens, legumes (lentils, chickpeas, pinto beans), and eggs. Look for methylfolate in your prenatal vitamins, which is the most absorbable form. You need 600 mcg of folate every day during your pregnancy.

Choline	Helps produce the neurotransmitter acetylcholine, which is essential for memory, mood, muscle control, and other nervous system functions	Eggs (include the yolk!), beef liver, pinto beans, brussels sprouts, quinoa, almonds, and tofu. You need 450 mg of choline daily.
Glycine	Needed to develop your baby's bones and teeth, internal organs, hair, skin, and nails	Bone broth, salmon, sesame seeds, pumpkin seeds, watercress, spirulina, spinach, and nori
Probiotics	Beneficial bacteria that keep mama's immune system and digestive system in check	Yogurt (check the label to make sure it contains *Lactobacillus bulgaricus*), kefir, aged cheese, miso, and other fermented foods like sauerkraut, pickles, and kimchi
Prebiotics	Fiber-rich foods that help "feed" the probiotics	Vegetables, berries, and oats

Sweet Potato Quiche

Ingredients

2 medium sweet potatoes, washed

Olive oil spray

Salt and pepper to taste

1 teaspoon extra-virgin olive oil

1/2 onion, chopped

2 big handfuls spinach

1 cup chopped broccoli florets

7 eggs, beaten

3 tablespoons water, milk, or almond milk

1/4 cup shredded mozzarella, optional

1. Preheat oven to 350°F.
2. Thinly slice your clean sweet potatoes. (Don't peel them, though. There are lots of nutrients in the skin.) These will be your "crust," so you'll want the slices to be as consistent as possible. I use a mandoline for speed and uniformity, but a knife is just fine.
3. Spray a pie dish with olive oil spray and line the dish with slices of sweet potato, starting at the bottom and then the sides, building your crust.
4. Once your crust is arranged, spray with olive oil spray, sprinkle with salt and pepper, and bake for 15 minutes.
5. While your crust is baking, heat 1 teaspoon of olive oil on the stove and sauté the onion, spinach, and broccoli. The more the merrier, so add in any of your favorite colorful veggies.
6. Whisk your eggs in a separate bowl and add water, milk, or almond milk (whatever you prefer).
7. When the crust is done, remove it from the oven and arrange your sautéed veggies in an even layer on the sweet potato crust. Pour the whisked eggs over the veggies and add some salt, pepper, and shredded cheese on top (that's optional, but delicious).
8. Bake for 25 to 30 minutes, or until the eggs are set. Let it stand for about 5 minutes before you dig in. Enjoy!

PS: Leftovers are amazing with a green salad for lunch or dinner.

Miso and Ginger-Glazed Salmon

Ingredients

2 (4-to-8-ounce) salmon filets
1 tablespoon freshly grated ginger

3 garlic cloves, minced

2 tablespoons miso paste

1 tablespoon tamari / soy sauce / coconut aminos

1 teaspoon toasted sesame oil

1 teaspoon sambal oelek, optional

1 tablespoon sesame seeds

Green onions (sliced) for garnish

1. Preheat oven to 425°F.
2. Line up your salmon filets on a baking dish or sheet pan lined with parchment paper.
3. To make the marinade, mix together the ginger, cloves, miso paste, tamari / soy sauce / coconut aminos, sesame oil, and the sambal oelek, and pour the mixture over the salmon. (You can use a silicone brush if you want to be fancy.) Add a sprinkle of sesame seeds on top.
4. Bake for 8 to 12 minutes, depending on how you like your salmon cooked.
5. Garnish with green onions and any leftover marinade.

PS: I like to pair the salmon with rice and a salad made of thinly sliced radishes, kale, and brussels sprouts.

FIVE

THE HARD STUFF

One Saturday morning, right after I changed out of my pajamas and put on full glam to shoot my podcast, I put up a TikTok video and asked people what they wish they'd known about pregnancy. There were a lot of funny comments, but a lot of women gave me answers that were a lot tougher to talk about . . . which means we absolutely need to talk about them: pregnancy loss and infertility. I promised you I'd keep it real, and real life has a lot of hard stuff in it. This chapter is for the women going *through* this stuff and for the people who want to support you through it. If you need to rip this chapter out and mail it to the people who need to read it, you have my full permission to do it. If you need to skip this chapter because you just don't want this stuff in your headspace, that's totally fine. I feel you, bish. You can always flip back when and if you're ever ready for it. It's a book, it's not going anywhere!

PREGNANCY LOSS

Seeing that positive pregnancy test sent a jolt of joy through my body, followed by a rush of fear. I was pregnant, but would I *stay* pregnant?

The facts are that 10 to 25 percent of known pregnancies end in a miscarriage, meaning a pregnancy that ends on its own during the first twenty weeks of gestation.[1] The word *known* is key because 50 to 75 percent of miscarriages happen before a woman even knows she's pregnant.[2] But I did know that I was pregnant, and I was terrified. Miscarriages are most likely to happen in the first twelve weeks of pregnancy,[3] so the first trimester I felt like I was holding my breath, waiting to reach the magical twelve-week number where everything would be smooth sailing. I couldn't feel a bump, but every night I rubbed my lower belly and uterus and said, "Please stay with us," hoping to let this baby know how much we wanted them, how we were waiting for them, how they were already a part of our family.

Then one morning I wiped and saw dark blood. We'd had sex the night before and I totally freaked out. I was already terrified to have sex while pregnant. I couldn't not think, *Daryl's gonna poke the baby!* (It doesn't work like that.) I texted a picture of the blood to my doctor. It was fine, but every time I wiped after that incident, I checked for blood. A little spotting can be normal early in pregnancy, but it could also be a sign of miscarriage. Miscarriage symptoms are like a period: cramping, lower back pain, bleeding.[4] This is a total mindfuck because when you're already nervous (and I was), you feel like everything is a symptom. So you know I was already texting my doctor every paranoid thought about every little thing I *thought* I felt. And I wasn't embarrassed either. If you have any concern at all, call your provider. They probably have a twenty-four-hour nurse line, and they can talk you through what you're experiencing and help you decide whether you should come in.

It's hard for doctors to determine *why* a pregnancy ends in miscarriage, but during the first trimester, it's often a result of chromosomal abnormality.[5] Your provider will be able to guide you through the loss of your pregnancy, and a lot of women miscarry at home: you go home, have cramps and contractions, and "pass" (ick, what an awful medical term) all the tissue and blood. If it sounds horrible . . . yeah, it's pretty horrible. Some women may be eligible for a D&C—a dilation and curettage—to complete the miscarriage and heal properly. It's an outpatient medical procedure that I won't describe in detail. Some women *need* it, but others opt in to avoid having to go home and pass the tissue and embryo or fetus on their own. You already know that one of the rules of this book is no judgment, and this applies triple here: we aren't going to judge ourselves or other mamas for how they get through this kind of thing. Talk to your doctor and do what you gotta do.

What I want you to know is that it's not your fault. It didn't happen because you went on a jog or because you took a sip of champagne before you knew you were pregnant. It didn't happen because you weren't grateful enough or because you forgot to take your vitamins. You do not need to blame yourself or pick apart everything you did—or didn't do—in the days and weeks before this loss. This is not something I've experienced, but because it *is* common, I've asked women I know who *have* experienced pregnancy loss for some advice.

Taking Care of Yourself After Pregnancy Loss

This loss is also your story to tell, and you get to decide who knows about it and how they get that information. If you're a private person who just needs the support of your partner and closest family members, you have the right to say, "This loss is very personal, and I'd appreciate it if you keep this information between us. I will tell people when and if I decide to do that." If you need the support of a wider community, you have the right to put this on social media, send an email, or shout it from the rooftop (just, be safe, roofs are pretty high). Anyone who judges you for talking about your loss is not your friend, and that's facts. They suck.

Grieve the loss. Pregnancy loss is a normal, natural part of the pregnancy process, but that doesn't mean it's not heartbreaking. Women who miscarry have heard things like "Well, at least you know you can get pregnant" or "At least it happened early," and I would not blame you for wanting to slap anyone who says this kind of shit to you. You wanted that baby, and now it's gone. Please do not let anyone tell you how you should feel or how you should react to that loss. Cry it out, rage it out, fill up your journal, pray. There's no getting around grief; there is just going through it. Take your time, bestie.

Be honest. People can't help but ask how you're doing, even though the answer should be pretty obvious. Tell your people the truth, even if you're afraid it will make them uncomfortable. Tell them if you're heartbroken, if you're numb, if you're actually okay. They're not asking to be annoying (even if it's annoying); they're asking because they want to know. And if they can't handle the truth, well, they should have asked you about the weather. Period.

Get whatever help you need. You might not know what help you need, but try a lot of things. Get a therapist if you don't have one already. Therapy is not cheap here in the US, but there are a lot of online options now that make it more affordable *and* mean you don't have to drive a half hour, sit awkwardly in a waiting room, and then look around the room for tissues. You can be in your own house and have your own tissues ready. I'm willing to bet that you have friends and family who have been through pregnancy loss and are willing to walk through it with you, and if you don't: get online and find your people. There are support groups and Facebook groups and Reddit communities filled with women supporting one another through this loss. You might feel lonely, but you're not alone in this pain.

Doctor's Note

Part of my job is being with women for their highs *and* lows, and one of those lows is miscarriage. While it's very common, it doesn't make it hurt any less. What I want all my patients—and you—to know is that it is nothing you did, didn't do, should have done, or could have done. It is not your fault. Miscarriage is your body's way of protecting you from moving forward with a pregnancy that isn't healthy. Normalizing it is not meant to minimize the experience but to help you remember that you are absolutely not alone. Let yourself feel sad, and let yourself grieve. I've had patients say that they feel strange grieving for a baby that wasn't real . . . but your baby was real! It existed inside you and in the future you imagined as a family. Don't rush yourself to feel better, but know that the majority of women who experience miscarriage go on to have healthy pregnancies. When patients ask, "When can I try again?" I tell them they can try when they feel physically *and* emotionally ready.

How to Be a Good Friend to a Person Who Miscarried

Here's why I love my friends: we keep each other's deepest, darkest secrets; we pick lettuce out of each other's teeth; we hold each other's hair back after a rough night. I think most of us want to be the best possible friend we can: we want to be the kind of girl someone can lean on when things are hard. And again, statistically, most of us are going to be supporting a friend through pregnancy loss at some point. It's horrible to think of, I know, but I'm a woman who likes to be prepared, so as I mentioned, I asked some friends about how their friends and family best supported them through their miscarriages.

First things first: you need to show up. Ummm, kind of obvious, I know, but I heard from lots of women that when they lost their baby, they were surprised at who *didn't* show up. Pandemic aside, these women were alone in their grief and their loss, except for maybe a text here or there. A part of me does get it: nobody wants to intrude, and nobody wants to say the wrong thing. I've put my foot in my mouth enough times to know that it doesn't taste good, but I've learned it's enough to say, "I'm sorry. I don't know what to say, but I love you and

I'm here for you." Text it; call it; write it in a letter. Do all of the above, and do it even when she doesn't reply. In fact, let her know that she doesn't *need* to reply, that you love her no matter what.

Everyone I asked told me that the worst thing in the world is hearing "Let me know what I can do." Nobody wants to sit around thinking of a job for you to do, girl! Just pick a thing and do it. Drop a meal off at her doorstep; send her your favorite candle; get her a massage at her very favorite spa. One friend shared with me:

> I was too sad to even think straight after my miscarriage, but my friend texted me every few days with options: Would I like a homemade dinner dropped off for my family, or DoorDash from my favorite restaurant? Would it be helpful to take my older kids for two hours on Thursday night, or for a few hours on Saturday? Would I like some company and *Real Housewives* on the couch, or to be alone tonight? I couldn't have thought of a single thing if she'd asked me what I needed, but I could always choose between a few good options, and I never felt pressured to say yes to anything just to make her feel better.

But, Meghan, what if I'm *pregnant? Won't showing up with my big ol' pregnant belly make her sad?* I don't know. Friendships are like any long-term relationship; they take a lot of communication. If you're pregnant and your friend *isn't* pregnant anymore, don't assume that the sight of you is going to drive her into a depression; *ask her how she feels about it.* Let her know that you want to be sensitive to her loss and that she has the option of seeing or hearing about your pregnancy *if she is open to it.* Let her know it's okay to mute you on social media if she needs to and that she can change her mind at any time. Another friend recalled:

> My best friend and I got pregnant at the same time and had our first babies just months apart. And then got pregnant *again* at

the same time . . . except that I miscarried just before the twelve-week mark, before we'd told each other. When I told her about my miscarriage, she *didn't* tell me about her pregnancy. I found out when she was about four months along, and my heart broke: I was so happy for her, and I hated that she had been afraid to tell me. Yes, I was sad for my loss, but I didn't want her to dim her joy for me. Her son was born two weeks after my baby was due, and he reminds me of everything good in this world.

Maybe the most genius piece of advice I heard was this: Use your calendar to help you be a better friend. Put her due date in your calendar and check in with her as it gets closer. How is she feeling? Does she want to talk about it? If the answer is no, that's *fine*, but at least you asked.

INFERTILITY

Getting pregnant was easy for me the first time, and while I'm writing this, I'm hoping it will come just as easily the second time too. But it's not easy for everyone. I have friends who struggled for years to conceive, and I know people who have gone nearly broke paying for fertility treatments. It's not a pain I understand (knock on wood), but I get why they do it: when you want a child, you *want a child*. You want a child so badly that you'd do anything to get that child. You already know I put a DivaCup inside me to catch as many sperm as possible; you think I wouldn't go to the ends of the earth to have a baby? If you told me I had to hang upside down by my ankles for an hour, or spend all the money in my bank account, I'd do it.

When Is It Officially Infertility?

According to the American College of Obstetricians and Gynecologists, couples who haven't gotten pregnant after trying for a year without any birth control should go get an evaluation. If you're older than thirty-five, they suggest an evaluation after six months.[6] I'd have been beating down the door of the doctor's office after three months, max, but you already know how I am. Before you freak out, just talk to your provider and take it one step at a time.

Doctor's Note

I'm not a reproductive specialist, but I know how scary and frustrating the conception process can be for many women and couples. If my patient is over forty and hasn't gotten pregnant after a few months of trying, I suggest they see a specialist. If they're younger than thirty-five, I tell them to try for a year. Half of those couples will be pregnant in six months, and 90 percent of them will be pregnant in a year, and it doesn't do any good to stress about it because even stress can make it harder to conceive. If you're a person who is comforted by knowing as much as you can, there's no harm in seeing a specialist to get as much information and education about your fertility as possible to make informed decisions about your family planning.

For worriers like me, here's how fertility evaluations generally go:

Men have to go jerk off into a cup somewhere to have their sperm looked at. And I've heard it's a small, sad room, so *bring your phone, men!* They're looking at how many swimmers they have, how well they swim, and how they're shaped. Your guy *might* have to get a scrotum ultrasound or something more invasive, but first things first: he has to go do something he's been doing regularly since middle school. Poor guy.

You'll both answer questions about your medical history, your family's medical history, your medications. Future mamas will talk about their periods and their reproductive health in general and may have to give some blood and urine. Your doctor will either refer you to a specialist or run some more tests, and they'll all do their best to try to solve the puzzle with you. There's no book and no website and for sure no YouTube video that can diagnose you or tell you why it's not working the way you want it to. But I don't blame you if you want to go nuts and search for every possible outcome. I would definitely be doing that.

Some Infertility Treatment Options

You know what sucks even worse about infertility? How expensive it is! Many insurance companies don't cover infertility treatments. The costs vary, depending on your medical coverage, and the value of the treatment depends on your own financial situation and your definition of expensive, but my jaw hit the *floor* when I learned about how expensive it can be to build a family.

What It's Called	What It Is	What It Costs
Intrauterine insemination (IUI)	A provider takes the sperm and, ya know, puts it in you. There's more to it than that: the sperm is washed and concentrated so you're getting the best of the best, and it's injected into you when you're ovulating. Your doctor might monitor your ovulation and might give you medication to get you to release more eggs at the ideal time. The actual insemination takes place at the doctor's office and takes less than a half hour: you put your feet in the stirrups, spread your legs, and stare at the ceiling while a doctor or nurse inserts a long, thin tube into your vagina and right up through the cervical opening into the uterus so the sperm can go catch an egg, fast.[7] My friend's doctor set an egg timer for fifteen minutes afterward, and then my friend went back to work like it hadn't been the weirdest lunch hour ever.	$$

In vitro fertilization (IVF)	IVF is the process of taking sperm and eggs to create embryos that can be implanted in the uterus. This all happens in a laboratory, obviously, and involves stimulating ovulation, retrieving the eggs, getting sperm from the man (again, they really have it easy in these scenarios), and fertilizing the eggs with those sperm. Healthy embryos are then implanted right into the uterus, and the two-week wait begins. Some couples need donor sperm and/or eggs to do this, which of course costs more money.	$$$$
Gestational surrogacy	Some couples need a woman to carry the pregnancy for them. Gestational surrogates have a couple's fertilized embryos implanted in them via IVF. They aren't a genetic parent, but they take on the entire process of pregnancy and birth on behalf of the parents.	$$$$$

Help, I Need Support!

You can find support groups all over the United States at resolve.org, the website for the National Infertility Association. But you may also want support from family and friends, which means you'll have to tell them. This sucks, because shouldn't the people who love us just know what we need without being told? Yeah, they should be able to read our minds, but unfortunately, that is not currently possible. So even though you're the person who is struggling right now, it's still on you to let people know.

I'm a trauma dumper. I tell everyone everything. It's really tempting to just dump all your trauma in a text message or a phone call, but before you do that, check in with the person you want support from. Ask, "Can I talk to you about something hard?" Trust that if they say yes, they mean it, and if they say it's not a good time for them, that it's not personal (that part is hard when you're *personally* going through something). Experiencing infertility can mean hurting for an indefinite period of time. Your feelings about this experience might change, and what you need from those around you might change too. In the thick of it, you might not know what you need—that's understandable—but as much as possible, be specific with the people around you. If you need your people to listen while you vent, or help you find solutions, or offer advice, tell them. I find that communication in *all* my relationships is the key to life. And if there's something that absolutely *doesn't* help, tell them! I say this from the outside looking in on this experience: the people around you feel just as helpless as you do, and everyone wants to show up for you in the right way. But at some point they're absolutely going to say and do the wrong thing.

A Few Ways to Ask for What You Need

- I'm feeling really sad. Do you have the capacity to listen to me vent?
- I don't know what to do next. Do you have any insights you could share with me?
- I have an appointment on Wednesday and I'm anxious. Could you come over the night before to distract me?
- I know you care about me and want to help, but texting me articles about possible infertility treatments makes me feel overwhelmed. Can we avoid that topic over text message?

There's enough to say about this topic to fill a million books, so let me end by saying this: I see you, I hear you, and I'm so sorry this is happening. I wish you all the happy, healthy babies your heart desires, and I'm rooting for you.

How to Be a Good Friend to Someone Struggling with Infertility

If I could, I would grant every person on Earth the ability to have the babies they are aching for. I'm sorry if your road to motherhood was a long one, or if you're still hoping to step on the path. I'm sorry if you've experienced this kind of pain and if you're trying to help another person through it. Words alone can't fix it, but words are a huge part of how we connect with one another. I write songs (and now, books! She does it all) about human connection, and I still find it difficult to find the right words when friends are struggling to get pregnant, especially since Riley came so easily to me. I feel a little guilty. But that's putting my own feelings at the center of this experience that isn't mine, and I have to remind myself that this is *not about me.* I don't need to offer advice unless I'm asked for it; I don't need to fix things; I just need to be there to *listen.*

WHAT NOT TO SAY

Everything happens for a reason!
Why don't you just adopt?
Have you tried [insert very personal medical choice here]?
Have you tried [insert something you saw on YouTube here]?

The women I know who have struggled with infertility have also struggled to find a way to talk about it with the people they love. Not everyone is comfortable with everyone knowing their business (can't relate, but I get it). And some people *want* to talk about it but don't want to make other people uncomfortable. They don't want their friends to feel bad for getting pregnant; they don't want people to worry about them; they don't want to ruin the vibe at the dinner party. I never want someone I love to feel like they have to hide their pain from me, and if I were going through infertility, I *promise* you I'd never shut up about it. You'd all have to hear about my IVF, my embryos, all of it. Your support is only as good as the information you have, so here are some questions that might get you the answers you need to be the best supporter you can:

- Is this something you want to talk about with me?
- Do you want me to ask about it, or would you prefer to give updates when you're comfortable?
- Are you comfortable with hearing about my own fertility and pregnancy journey? It's cool if you're not.
- Is it helpful to hear about what worked for me? If not, I can STFU.
- If I say or do the wrong thing, please let me know. I got you, girl.

Ask questions and pay attention to the answers. If you're offering to listen, you need to actually listen. If you say you're open to feedback, you have to apologize when you do or say the wrong thing (even when it's unintentional). Friendships don't always get the same celebration as our romantic partnerships, but we need one another—especially when stuff gets hard. I had a conversation with Dr. Drew Pinsky on my podcast *Workin' On It*, and he said the most beautiful thing: "Brains heal other brains."[8] We literally need one another, so let your friends know right now that you have their backs.

PART TWO

TRIMESTER TWO

SIX

TWELVE WEEKS

Girl, you made it. At twelve weeks, the first trimester is officially over. The apps told me that at this point, my baby was starting to actually look like a baby. A little, lime-sized baby with a face and fingers and all that good stuff. I still didn't have a bump, just a constant bloat as if I ate a fat burrito every day, which kept convincing me there was no baby and I'd made it up. "Yes, there's a baby in there!" Daryl would assure me. I don't know why he was so sure . . . maybe because my boobs were getting huge? I didn't really *have* the symptoms that women complain about, but the apps told me that if I *was* exhausted or nauseous, that was about to get a lot better. But the twelve-week mark felt like a big deal because the risk of miscarriage drops significantly, and I finally felt myself take a breath.

YOUR PREGNANCY, YOUR NEWS

Your pregnancy is your news to share, and you get to decide how and when to tell people. There's no rule that says you have to wait until twelve weeks, and there's no rule that says you have to make exceptions for the people in your life who would want to know earlier. For me, it felt right for my parents and brothers to be the first people to hear about the pregnancy, followed by my closest friends and my team (who are all like family to me), and then my extended family . . . and then every single person I crossed paths with. But I also think that having a front-row seat into a person's life is a privilege, and you get to decide who earned it.

A lot of people don't tell anyone but their partner and their provider about the pregnancy until they hit the twelve-week mark, so the end of the first trimester also means throwing open the windows and letting the world in on your good news. If you're feeling highly emotional, I do *not* recommend going on YouTube and watching pregnancy announcement videos. But if you want a good cry? They are the best videos ever. There are probably tens of thousands of videos of people finding out they're going to be a grandparent or a parent for the first time, that magical moment when they find out that their whole world is about to change. I watched tons of these before I even got pregnant, and I thought about how I'd tell Daryl. Maybe I'd get a tiny Spy Kid outfit and have him unwrap it. Maybe I'd write a song and sing it to him. Obviously, you know how that turned out.

And once I knew, I had absolutely zero chill and zero interest in taking the time to think about how to tell my parents in the most dazzling way possible. I was pregnant, I was thrilled, and I just wanted to *tell* them, like right away. So Daryl and I drove on over to my parents' house. I was out of the car before it was fully in Park, barging into the kitchen and whipping out my positive pee stick. YouTube had prepared me for a big, emotional moment, but y'all, this is the Trainor family, and my dad always wants to make a funny in every situation, even when it's a positive, life-changing one. That's why we love him . . .

the dad jokes. So no, he didn't crumple into a crying mess; he looked at the test, looked up at me, and said with a straight face, "It's the beginning of the end." *Dad!*

We all laughed uncomfortably, but my mom was smiling like crazy. "Does it really say pregnant?" she asked, looking at the test again and again.

"*Yas! I'm pregnant!*" I screamed.

To be fair, they probably weren't shocked, because I announced to the entire family when we were trying and told them the specific days we were trying. I'm obnoxious.

We were all laughing and hugging, and no, it wouldn't have made for good YouTube content, but it was accurate and perfect for my adorable, loving parents.

If you think you have to go all out for your pregnancy announcements, I can tell you right now that people will be just as excited and joyful hearing it in casual conversation as they would be if you went all out. There's just something about knowing that a baby is on the way that makes everyone feel happy, no production value required.

I was pregnant during the height of COVID-19, and I was also producing a Christmas album. I had to tell everyone in the studio to make sure they took the testing and protocols seriously.

I'm a bigmouth, but I also like to be able to tell people my own news; it sucks to feel like you're sharing something big with another person only to have them say, "Oh, I know, I heard."

IT'S A GIRL! I THINK. I'M CERTAIN. I THINK.

For us, the twelve-week mark was important for another reason: we'd finally get the results of our blood test back and know the sex of our baby. Some people don't find out until the twenty-week ultrasound, but do you think I could wait that long? Hell no. Some people don't find out until the baby is *born*, and to them I say, How do you live with that kind of suspense?!

I didn't think we needed the test because I was already 100 percent sure I was having a girl. When the apps told me that my baby was the size of a blueberry, I knew that my blueberry had long blond hair and could *sing* and we would be best friends, just like me and my mom. Back when I was spreading the news to anyone with ears, I didn't just say, "I'm pregnant." I said, "I'm pregnant and it's a girl. Potentially twins." Nobody—not a single soul—had told me I was having twins, but I said this as though it was an absolute fact. It felt like a fact because YouTube was filled with all these old wives' tales about what a "girl pregnancy" feels like: Pregnancy acne? Check. Craving sweets? Sure. Morning sickness? Okay, no, but it didn't matter: it was a girl, and the blood test was just a way to confirm how correct I was.

But *still*. The day we knew we'd get the results, my heart was racing. I kept walking around the house, saying to Daryl, "Today we find out about our girrrrrl!" I watched my phone like a hawk and checked at least one hundred times to make sure the ringer was on. And then it rang. Daryl and I held hands while the nurse told us, "Actually, it's a boy."

A boy?! A boy! I put my head in my hands and started crying. Not sad tears. Happy tears. It was like being told I was pregnant all over again but even better because I could actually start picturing my baby. I could just see him: red hair and big eyes and a kind heart, just like his dad. He'd be funny and silly and sweet.

Daryl Says

As a rule, I always want what Meghan wants, so I was Team Girl all the way. And as much as I'd love a little Meghan someday, I was relieved to know our first baby would be a boy. Maybe it's because

I'm a guy, and I felt like it would be easier for me? I laugh at that now, because I *still* didn't have a clue when Riley was born. And after Riley, I'm just stoked to make as many babies as we can.

But under my happy tears there was something else . . . something I categorized as a demon thought, something I couldn't tell anyone and would have to take to the grave with me: I was bummed, y'all. Not majorly bummed, but I was disappointed. I had already spent all that time imagining my little girl, and I was attached to her. I wanted to brush her hair and teach her to sing and watch her do little performances in the living room like I was always doing with my family. The minute I heard "It's a boy," all those little moments just—*poof!*—disappeared. There was no little girl. I'd still be the only girl, stuck in a house full of boys. (My two brothers live in our house with us.) I know we're all supposed to just be amped to have a healthy, happy baby—and we were!—but I just want to say for any other moms out there who have all their eggs in one basket . . . it's okay to be a little disappointed if you don't get what you were expecting. You're not a monster. You're not ungrateful. You just spent a few weeks in your own imagination, building a relationship with a version of your baby who doesn't exist. I wasn't walking around the house sulking, but a part of my heart felt a little sad that I was wrong. Plus, I mean, I'd already told so many people I was *for sure* having a girl. Embarrassing!

Once I let go of the momentary disappointment of knowing that I wasn't having a little version of me, I was *pumped* for this boy. I could imagine him with more detail every day. I practiced saying "our son" and smiled like a goofball. I imagined him in little matching outfits with Daryl, dressing him up for Halloween, him playing video games with my brothers. I am the only girl in my family, and my brothers are literally my best friends (usually), so the more I got used to the idea, the more it started to feel like destiny.

I wanted to do a gender reveal so badly, but as we all know, I also have zero patience. So instead I did individual gender reveals that were absolutely not Pinterest-worthy in any way. I turned on the video on my phone and made people guess what we were having. I started with my brothers and my uncle Steve, and each of them said the same thing: "Well, you're smiling, so it must be a girl." Before they were even done saying the word "girl," Daryl and I were shouting *"It's a boy!"* In all our lives, I have never seen that much pure joy on my brothers' faces. I know they'd have been happy either way, but hearing they were getting another little guy to add to their pack definitely had them stoked. That got me even more stoked. We were having a boy!

YOUR BABY, YOUR BOUNDARIES

Once people know you're pregnant, get ready to be showered with love, attention, and . . . questions. I've always known that people are curious, but pregnancy taught me that people are nosy as hell! Personally, I'm an open book and a borderline oversharer, but not everyone wants to get into a conversation about breastfeeding with a stranger at the pharmacy. And you shouldn't have to! There's something about a pregnant belly that makes people lose their minds and any sense of boundaries. Name another time in a woman's life where a person would randomly try to rub her belly. Wouldn't happen.

Pregnant women are subject to all kinds of questions: Are you going to find out the gender? What names are you considering? Are you going to stay at home or go back to work? What's your birth plan? How's your cervix feeling? What are you craving? Personally, I think you have the right to tell anyone to mind their business, but if you want some more socially acceptable ways to say "back the fuck off," here are some options:

- I'm not comfortable talking about that with anyone but my partner or my doctor.
- We aren't sharing our baby's name until they've arrived.
- Thanks for asking, but I don't want to discuss that right now.

If you're nervous to say any of these (people pleaser over here!), try it with a smile to soften the blow.

MAMA'S SECOND-TRIMESTER PERMISSION SLIP

By the end of your second trimester, your hormones are going buck wild. Your internal organs have rearranged themselves to accommodate a whole-ass person that you grew inside of you. Hello, you made a skeleton! Teeth! A tiny little heart! Fingers! Toes! Balls! Or extra ovaries! And you did all that while you were also doing whatever your other jobs are. You are probably wondering how the hell you are gonna get even bigger and how your ankles won't break under you. You might be realizing that this baby has to come out of you somehow and you are freaking out. These are all valid and normal feelings. Just in case you need a little reminder, this and so much more has earned you permission to do whatever the heck you want, including but not limited to:

- Crying whenever you want, especially if it's a YouTube pregnancy reveal for a couple who has been trying for years.
- Giving up on cute maternity clothes and wearing only your husband's giant sweatshirts and whatever leggings you can get over your belly. Actually, fuck it, you can just roll those leggings under the belly if you have to.
- Thinking *That's the dumbest thing I've ever heard* when a complete stranger gives you unsolicited advice on how to be pregnant. Some people just weren't born with the ability to

realize when they're overstepping their bounds, bless their hearts.

- Questioning your husband's taste and honesty when he says you've never looked more beautiful. *Like, never-never, buddy? Really? Don't you think that's a little insulting to the version of me that showed up looking like a real-life princess at our wedding?* I'm mostly joking, but damn.
- Having a full-on meltdown when you face a minor inconvenience. There's just a lot going on inside you right now, and you can't always keep it together when the one snack you were looking forward to all day is mysteriously missing from the fridge and your husband and brothers are all pointing the finger at one another. (Is that just a me thing?)
- Prioritizing yourself and your health above everything else. Canceling plans last minute can be a mama's best friend.
- Documenting your body. Your body is beautiful, even if you don't think so right now. This is a moment in time, and if you're miserable right now, having photos to look back at will remind you that you *were* beautiful. I'm lucky I have a full-on team for glam, but a girl at the makeup counter at the mall can make you pretty. You don't need to hire a fancy photographer if money is tight; my *brother* took my maternity pictures. I don't recommend this, because my nips were slipping and I'm pretty sure he's traumatized . . . but put on some makeup and have your girlfriend or husband take some photos. This moment will pass, and it's worth documenting.

SEVEN

MENTAL HEALTH IS HEALTH

Like a lot of moms, I was anxious about being pregnant. But like a lot of people, I was anxious wayyyyyy before I ever got pregnant. For some people, anxiety is a passing emotion or a temporary reaction. But I've been an anxious creature for as long as I can remember.

Middle children get a bad rap for being trouble, but I *was* the problem child. I had a lot of outbursts. My mom can laugh about it now, but it couldn't have been easy to have a little girl freaking the hell out because the volume indicator lines on the car's LED screen weren't even, or because her big brother was scratching the fabric of the car roof by her head. (But seriously, Ryan, WTF. Why did you torture me?) I have the *best* family, but just imagine being around a little girl who needs to hum after every single sip of liquid. That was me every time I took a sip of a drink: I'd *have* to make a little humming noise every time. Not just one little-cute-melody hum, but an even-number-of-chants hum: four or eight or ten.

If you're thinking, *Damn, Meghan, this sounds like OCD . . .* you're correct! It was! My OCD was lit. Still is. My brothers and parents sat through probably thousands of meals like this—and you all know I love the hell out of my brothers, but they *ridiculed* me for this. I felt like a weirdo and a freak.

And *then* . . . I started picking and peeling. This might be the grossest part of the book (until we get to childbirth), but it started with picking the skin on my fingers. You might be thinking about little hangnails or messy cuticles . . . no. And I've never told anyone this publicly, so we are really getting into my secrets, but I would use a nail clipper and peel the entire skin off my thumbs like a snake shedding its skin. I know, I know. But I get the same satisfaction that some people might get from biting their nails off. This is my vice. It's like successfully popping a huge pimple. When I'm done it feels like, "New skin, new me!"

As a kid, I thought I was 100 percent the grossest weirdo in the world, but we know a lot more about mental health than we did in the 2000s, and I have a therapist who has reassured me that actually, the world is filled with people whose brains are as *unique* as mine. One doctor told me it was my way of comforting myself, almost like rubbing my own back. My uncle peels his fingers just like I do! And even though I've had these compulsions since childhood, I was *mostly* okay. Aside from the humming and the peeling and the other secret compulsions, most of my childhood was what I would call "soft anxiousness," a general sort of anxiety about everything and nothing.

And *then*, in 2014, my life turned upside down in the best way. I was just nineteen when "All About That Bass" broke through and became a megahit. I went from being a teenage girl in Nantucket to having everyone in the world singing my song, from living in my parents' house to living out of suitcases and hotel rooms. *I won a freaking Grammy.* It was everything I ever dreamed of, and it was . . . a lot. I'd wake up in the morning unsure of what city I was even in and fall asleep in a different time zone that night. I coped by self-medicating with weed. I couldn't *smoke* it, but I could have edibles, and getting a little (or a lot) high helped me get out of my head and my body and just *exist*. It was like when I was high, I wasn't a "famous person" anymore; I was just a person. That worked until it didn't.

It was 4 a.m. in New York City, and I was in glam getting ready to announce the 2016 Grammy nominations. I'd won a Grammy the year before, and it was a privilege to announce the following year's nominees alongside the iconic Gayle King. I also knew I needed vocal surgery, which was necessary for me to keep my career—and would also interrupt it. My bestie/assistant Jojo was running through the schedule for the week while I was in hair and makeup. She listed off dozens of meetings, flights, interviews, performances, deadlines, and it all started to blur together in my brain.

"How?" I asked. "How will I do all that?"

I'd been doing *all that* for years, not just as a pop star but as a songwriter hustling her ass off, but suddenly, I couldn't do it. I couldn't even *think* about doing it. I couldn't breathe. I started crying. I was having my first panic attack. I didn't know that, but Jojo and Daryl knew exactly what was happening.

Jojo told me to call out the objects in the hotel room, and I sat there saying, "Bed, phone, carpet . . ." I calmed down enough to get through the live TV appearance next to Gayle King. But I was freaked out. I'd never felt so out of control of my mind and my body, and even though I doubt anyone watching could tell, the Meghan who was reading out the names of the Grammy nominees was just an autopilot version of me, waiting to fall back into the icy waters of hell.

I am used to keeping my shit *together*—I pride myself on being early for meetings, making deadlines, being a boss—but I was falling apart. When the camera was off, my body was still vibrating, and the second panic attack was setting in. I was supposed to be heading to another interview, but my team saw my pale face and glassy eyes and knew I had to cancel everything on my schedule and go home. But I didn't just need a break; I needed help.

Did I get it right away? Of course not! I spent four months in hell, cycling in and out of panic attacks and feeling like I was losing my mind because I would fully dissociate from my body when people were speaking to me, or feel my throat close as I was falling asleep at night, or see things move that Daryl assured me were not moving. When I wasn't having a panic attack, I was beating myself up because here I was crying hysterically and struggling to breathe when I had everything I had ever wanted: dream career, dream guy, dream life. But it turns out even if your life is great, your brain chemicals don't really care. And I wanted it to be literally anything else! Even when Daryl was like, "Babe, these are panic attacks," I would be like, "Nahhhhhh, I think it's something else." I straight up went to the emergency room and told the doctors that I was having *an allergic reaction to steak* when I started to lose it after dinner one night. Had I ever been "allergic to steak" before? Absolutely not. Was I? Nope. It was a panic attack!

I just didn't understand that our minds can have that kind of effect on our bodies. It took me months to see a psychiatrist, and when I told him everything I was experiencing, I was sure that he would send me to an inpatient mental-health facility or, you know, tell me I was just allergic to steak. Instead, he told me in the calmest, most reassuring voice, "It sounds like you have panic disorder. Your chemicals are unbalanced, and we're going to balance them." I left that office with a diagnosis and a plan: 30 mg of citalopram, better known as Celexa. This tiny pill saved my ass, and after a month, the vibrations and torture finally stopped.

Why am I telling you all this? Because when my first OB referred to the medication that saved my life as "candies," he made me feel stupid and careless and insignificant. So I found myself a new doctor. Well, first I went to the car and cried, and then went home and cried to Daryl, and then I called some friends and cried, and then I talked with my psychiatrist, who told me that this doctor was being incredibly inappropriate and I should find another ob-gyn.

So I did. At sixteen weeks—after calling every powerful woman I know in Los Angeles for their recommendations—I walked into my first appointment with Dr. Solky. From the moment she walked into the room I felt calm and comfortable. We chatted through my family medical history, and she asked whether I was planning on a circumcision for the baby.

"Nah," I said. "I'd like to push him out if I can."

Apparently, I was thinking about the word *cesarean*, not about my baby's foreskin. I was mortified, but instead of making me feel like a dummy, she laughed in a way that made me feel totally not judged. When she told me there were no stupid questions, I believed her.

I learned from that first appointment with Dr. Solky that my standards were way too low. A doctor should make you feel seen and heard, should take the time to listen to you and ask questions, and should never make you feel stupid. I asked Dr. Solky about my medications and we talked it through. She assured me the baby would be fine with it and that a happy mom is a happy baby and to not change anything if it's working. I left that appointment wishing I'd been seeing Dr. Solky since day one.

Doctor's Note

One of the best parts of my job is the relationships that I build with my patients. I've delivered babies for patients I've been seeing since they were teenagers; I've held my patients' hands through pregnancy losses; I've been there for huge life milestones. I'm not the right doctor for *everyone*, but I'm the right doctor for my patients. Pregnancy is a big experience physically and emotionally, and the most important thing you can have with your doctor is trust. Trust is built—and broken—in a million different ways, but for me, I want my patients to feel comfortable asking—and telling—me anything. Even if it means confusing *circumcision* and *cesarean*.

Mothers have always been expected to put themselves last. I'm pretty sure that even though we always ate dinner together as a family, my mom served her kids and husband before she fixed her own plate. And the second I found out that I was pregnant, I really did feel like my body and my life were no longer just my own. But that doesn't mean that I didn't matter anymore. Moms matter. We're the reason people exist! Taking care of your mental health is just as important as taking care of your body with exercise and nutrition, and if you're struggling, you're absolutely not alone. (Your brain will tell you that you are alone; your brain is lying.) Between 14 and 23 percent of women will experience symptoms of depression while pregnant.[1] Look around your friend group or your prenatal classes; at least one of you is not feeling your best mentally, even though you're "supposed" to be over-the-moon happy.

If you're already on medication and are afraid to get pregnant: Talk to your provider and make a plan. Not all medications are safe for pregnancy, but you can't stop them cold turkey, and you might not have to. If your doctor is as rude as my first one was, kick them to the curb and find a provider who takes your mental health seriously.

If you're pregnant and starting to feel anxious or depressed: Tell someone! Your provider, your partner, your family (hopefully all of them). There is no shame in needing help and getting it.

If you can't afford to get help: First of all, it *should* be free. Mental health care in America is as bad as maternal health care, and that's saying something. The Affordable Care Act does require that all health plans provide some level of mental health coverage,[2] but it might not be much.

Your employer might offer counseling as a part of your employee assistance program (EAP), and telehealth services might be a good option for you too. *If you're in a mental health crisis in the United States, you can call or text 988 for immediate support.*

I get why people don't want to tell other people that they're struggling: they don't want to be judged or looked down on. And they shouldn't be! These issues are not a personal failure, and they don't have to be anyone's entire identity. Brains are complicated, and you can be experiencing depression and anxiety and still be a good mama-to-be. You can go to therapy and take medication and still be a capable mother. I still take medication, I see a therapist, and I am really intentional about my exercise habits and my nutrition, because when I feel good physically, I feel better mentally. It's taken me twenty-seven years to find the right combination of treatments, and I'm very privileged to have the access that I do.

The shame and stigma around mental health is bullshit, and it's not helping anyone if we force ourselves and other people to put on a happy face when our brains are telling us that everything is falling apart. You cannot just fake it till you make it, and if you struggled with any part of your mental health before getting pregnant, you have to raise your hand and get whatever help you can. And keep it raised after the baby arrives! Postpartum depression and anxiety can literally kill, and your baby and your family need you around. That's why I'll tell anyone and everyone that I'm a pop star and a mama with an anxiety disorder. I'll shout it from the rooftops (or to Hoda Kotb) so anyone who needs to hear this can hear it loud and clear: your mental health matters, and so do you.

EIGHT

BODY TALK

Y'all ready to get sexy? Because the second trimester was not sexy at all for me. I know I'm supposed to tell you what all the apps tell you: that my energy came back, that I was glowing, that I had never felt better in my body and I was a sensual fertility goddess. Uh, no.

I walked into the second trimester looking like a hot mess and feeling like a disaster. Inspiring, right?

Let's start from the top, specifically my face. I've always had pretty good skin, all things considered. I'll get a zit here and there, but I've never had bad acne. So when a bunch of red dots showed up all over my face, I thought, *What the fuck?* I ran my fingers over my face while staring at myself in the mirror. They didn't feel like zits, just dry little red dots, like someone had written on my face while I was sleeping. They were unpoppable, with no whiteheads in them (you know I tried). I racked my brain (and the internet) for answers: Had my makeup artist forgotten to disinfect their brushes? The dots were also dry . . . had I burned myself somehow? And they itched like crazy . . . was I allergic to something? I called my doctor to make an appointment and tried not to look in the mirror. I was four months along and starting to work on the promo for my Christmas album. This meant photo shoots, videos, you know, stuff you need your face for. I couldn't exactly be on screen itching my face off, and without makeup I looked like I was having middle school acne issues.

Turns out, I had a little something called *perioral dermatitis*. Sexy, right? It literally means "rash around the mouth," but I was lucky to have it around my nose, cheeks, and eyes too. I know, I'm special. Apparently, a lot of women get this during pregnancy (shout-out to everyone who chimed in on my TikTok video to let me know I was not alone), and some women get it even when they're not pregnant! We can blame hormones for that.

One of my new habits in the pandemic was TikTok. Okay, it's still TikTok. I love that app. But, y'all, I was getting *influenced* on there. Not just by everyone sharing their pregnancy stuff but by all the amazing beauty and skin-care creators. I'd see a video for a new foundation or a skin-care product and have it added to my cart before the video was even over. I'd fallen for one of those little skin vacuum things just a few weeks before—you know, the ones that have a "diamond tip" and promise to suck all the gunk out of your pores—and suddenly, my skin was raw and burnt, especially under my eyes. I stopped buying things off TikTok (not really, but I cooled it on the skin stuff), so basically I had to use antibiotics to keep my face from freaking out again.

Now let's move on down to the other sexy, exciting parts of the second trimester. By the twenty-week mark, you're not supposed to be sleeping on your back anymore.[1] There's a risk of cutting off a major blood vessel called the *vena cava*, so from here on out you're sleeping on your side. I was so worried I'd flip onto my back in the middle of the night that I spent every night sleeping on our couch, where the back of the couch could keep me from rolling over. You already know that Daryl—a prince, a *king*—spent every night out there with me. He'd also wake up in the middle of the night to me screaming, because I'd get crazy charley horses when I slept. It didn't matter how hydrated I was—and by this time I was carrying around a gallon water jug that, yes, I bought because of TikTok—my calves would cramp up in the middle of the night and I'd become the world's loudest alarm clock. Daryl would help me stretch out my calves, and I'd try to fall back asleep.

By the middle of the second trimester, I finally got my bump! Okay, it wasn't quite a bump-bump, but it was a start, and I was stoked.

The bump was hiding something that I was *not* stoked about: my stretch marks. Look, I know we're supposed to call them our "tiger stripes" and wear them as a badge of honor for the privilege of carrying our little angels into this world, but, *ladies*, my stretch marks *started at my vagine*. Yeah. You read that right. I didn't even see them at first, and Daryl kept that little detail to himself. But one day, when I was putting on deodorant, I started screaming for Daryl (this is a theme) and he ran in screaming "What?!" as if I'd fallen and broken something.

"Look at my arms!" I told him.

Red, squiggly stretch marks were creeping along my armpits. They weren't cute little pink stripes either. They were an angry purply-red, and they freaked me the hell out. I mean, stretch marks on your belly? Fine. Boobs? Makes sense. But what do my arms have to do with this?

Daryl did what Daryl always does, which is tell me that I'm hot and perfect. And I did what I always do: go online and do extensive research on how and why stretch marks happen. Soon every algorithm on my phone served me up ads for miracle creams. And. I. Bought. Them. All. All of them! I'd read that the most effective way to treat them was to use whatever product you were using every day, so I used *every* product *every* day. I was rubbing on oils and creams all damn day. I'm surprised Daryl could even hug me without me slipping through his arms, I was that lubed up. If YouTube had told me to fill my bathtub with mayonnaise and soak in it, I would have done that. Because I did not want these stretch marks! I was (and still am, TBH) struggling with my body image. I knew gaining weight was a part of my pregnancy, but, y'all, we all know that there is a difference between *saying* you're fine with it and *being* fine with it. I didn't feel a single kick until twenty-two weeks, and the internet kept telling me it was because of my thickness. It doesn't matter how much you love yourself; that's a hard thing to hear. Or read. Whatever. I had a lot of work to do on my self-perception and body positivity, but I just want to say for anyone else out there struggling to embrace all these sudden (and sometimes permanent) changes to their body: I get it.

I wasted a lot of money on stretch mark creams, by the way. Because they are a type of scar, nothing really gets rid of them, and it's not like you can prevent your skin from stretching, even if you're slapping on lotion three times a day like I was. Stretch marks are in my genes: my mom had them, her mom had them; there was nothing I could have done to keep from getting them, and nothing I could do to get rid of them either. They fade with time, and some products might make them get a little lighter or less pronounced, but only if you apply them *every single day for a long time*, and you're not going to get your skin back to the way it was, even if you get expensive treatments at the dermatologist.[2] The only oil that I truly saw make a difference was vitamin E oil, but this was after pregnancy when I wasn't really stretching anymore, so . . . maybe that's why? Use whatever makes you feel good, but keep your expectations low (and save your money!).

WEIRD STUFF YOUR BODY MIGHT DO

I was so frustrated about my perioral dermatitis because I'd never heard of this happening. This is why I'm always asking ladies about the weird stuff their bodies did during pregnancy, to see what else I don't know about. Like I said, I like to be prepared, and TikTok was happy to feed my curiosity by serving me up videos of women whose bodies had done things I hadn't even thought of yet. I'd save the video and bring it up to Dr. Solky at my appointments and she'd be like, "Yep, that happens." So here's a small sampling of the things I worried about that didn't happen to me—but could have. Pregnant bodies are amazing *and weird*, and if you ever feel like it's just you, know that there are a whole lot of women who are going through it with you.

- **Carpal tunnel syndrome.** (I thought you got that from typing too much?) Dr. Solky says: Swelling in your wrists (even if you can't see it) puts pressure on your nerves. Ouch!
- **Pemphigoid gestationis.** Basically, itchy plaque and fluid-filled blisters. Yikes!
- **Hyperemesis gravidarum.** This is like, extreme morning sickness that makes you throw up all the time. Very grateful I didn't go through this one.
- **Hemorrhoids.** Apparently this is super common during pregnancy. Lucky for Daryl, this wasn't me, or he'd have been taking care of it for me (lovingly, like he does everything).
- **Growing feet.** Your belly I get. But feet?? I saw a few women say that their feet grew one or two sizes . . . and stayed that way! I'd be pissed if my shoes didn't fit anymore.
- **Body hair.** Like, new hairs growing in places they didn't grow before. On your belly. Down your neck. Dr. Solky says: You'll grow a lot of hair . . . and then lose it!
- **Extreme heartburn.**
- **Gallstones.** No thank you!
- **Arthritis.** Why??
- **Melasma.** A (usually temporary) discoloration in your skin. Sometimes called "the mask of pregnancy," which makes it sound scary. It doesn't hurt you or the baby, and it usually goes away after pregnancy.
- **Skin tags in . . . weird places.** Dr. Solky says: Hormones! You might also see new moles or freckles.

- **Dark armpits.** Dr. Solky says: Blame the increase in estrogen! This is also why you may see a dark line from your pubic area to your belly button.
- **An actual human person coming out of you.** The wildest one of all. Truly bananas.

About Diastasis Recti with Rebecca ────────

Of the many, many changes your body goes through during pregnancy and postpartum, one of them is ab separation, also known as *diastasis recti*. This is when there is a partial or complete separation of your rectus abdominis muscles, which meet at the midline of your stomach. Diastasis recti happens along the midline, near the belly button. It appears as a gap or "pooch"; you may see that your belly is "coning" when you do a crunch. Diastasis recti can contribute to bloating, back pain, constipation, and a number of other things. Your provider will check for this at appointments, but here's an easy way to keep an eye on it yourself too:

1. Lie flat on your back, feet flat on the floor, knees bent. Bring your hands behind your head for support. Inhale and relax your belly.
2. On the exhale, lift your head and shoulders away from the ground slightly and engage your abdominal muscles like you would do in a crunch.
3. Look at your belly and with one hand, feel the midline of your stomach, around your belly button.
4. Use your fingertips to feel whether there is any separation along the midline. If the space between your rectus abdominis muscles at the midline is more than one or two fingers'-width apart, you may have diastasis recti.

Diastasis recti will often correct itself over time, but in some cases, it can last for months or even years or become permanent if it goes untreated. You can seek support by finding a trained physical or occupational therapist to aid in your recovery. If you get a C-section, you can ask your doctor to sew your abs back together. Meghan had that done!

NINE

SECOND-TRIMESTER FOOD AND FITNESS

Keep It Moving with Rebecca

Giving birth—however you do it—is a physical process, and in the second trimester we're going to take advantage of your renewed energy to build on your strength and endurance with a combination of cardio and strength exercises. The exercises below can be complemented with a nice walk: it's free, it's easy, and it's great cardio. You can continue the workouts you did preconception and during the first trimester—if they still feel good—but we're no longer doing any kind of jumping or any exercise that involves lying on your belly. As always, you're listening to your body and keeping your core tight.

Equipment Needed:

Dumbbells (5-to-8-pound weights or whatever you feel comfortable with)

Exercise mat

Box, bench, or chair

Your Affirmation:

My baby and I are growing together.

Second-Trimester Fitness

BELLY BREATHING

Do this as a warm-up or cooldown. Start on your hands and knees in a tabletop position with a neutral spine. Now imagine your belly is zipping up like a coat: start by tucking your hips and squeezing from your lower abs on up to your rib cage. When you're all zipped up, slowly release from your ribs back on down to your hips, ending in that neutral spine position. Repeat 5 to 10 times, focusing on slowly and intentionally tightening and releasing every muscle in your stomach.

Aim for 8 to 10 reps of each exercise, cycling through the set 3 times—unless your body tells you otherwise!

SET 1

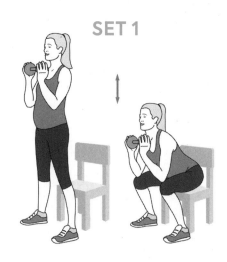

Dumbbell Box Squat

If you don't have a box, this works just fine with a dining chair. Start by standing in front of your box or chair, making sure it's not too low (for the right height, your legs should be at a 90-degree angle when you're sitting). Holding a dumbbell in front of your chest with both arms, squat down to a sitting position on the box/chair. Stand back up and repeat for additional reps. Keep your core engaged and make sure you're not leaning too far forward—your weight should stay in your heels, not your toes.

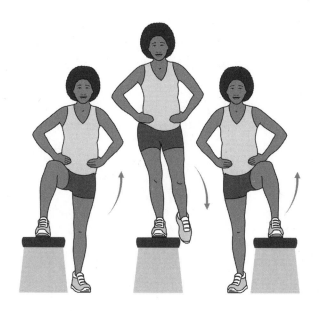

Bench Shuffles

Stand next to a low box or bench (12 inches or less), so your feet are parallel with the bench. With the foot closest to the bench, step up on to the bench and over to the other side. Go back and forth, only speeding up if you feel comfortable, to do a "shuffle" movement. Try this for 30 seconds without stopping.

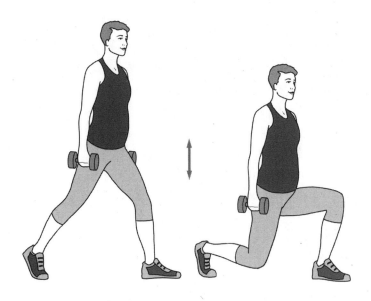

Stationary Lunge

Stand in a staggered stance / lunge position, holding your weights by your sides. Lower your body by bending your knees until they are both at a 90-degree angle. Don't worry about being geometrically perfect—just go as far down as your body allows you to go without pain or discomfort. Stand back up to your starting position and repeat for additional reps. After 8 to 10 reps, switch legs and repeat.

SET 2

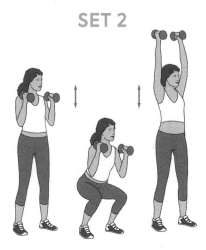

Dumbbell Squat to Press

Start with your feet shoulder-width apart, holding the dumb-bells up by your shoulders. Squat down (sitting on a box if needed), then stand back up. As you stand up, press the dumbbells overhead; lower them back down and repeat.

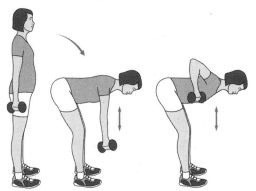

Dumbbell Deadlift Row

Start with your feet shoulder-width apart and your dumbbells down by your sides, palms facing each other. Hinge forward with your back straight and your core engaged, until your back is parallel with the floor. While you are in this position, pull the dumbbells up, leading with your elbows until your elbows are at a 90-degree angle by your sides. Lower dumbbells back down and stand straight up. Repeat for additional reps.

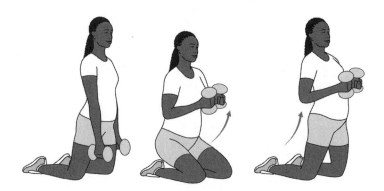

Kneeling Hip-Thrust Bicep Curl

Start with both knees on the floor, shoulder-width apart. With the dumbbells by your sides, palms facing in, raise them until your elbows are at a 90-degree angle. While the dumbbells are raised in a bicep-curl position, sit back on your heels and come back up, thrusting your hips forward. Lower dumbbells back down and repeat for additional reps.

Let's Eat with Kristy

We've all heard it—when you're pregnant, you're eating for two! That's true in the sense that your nutrition is your baby's nutrition, but it doesn't mean you're required to eat twice as much. And the real truth is that you only need to eat *more* starting now, in the second trimester, and only an additional three hundred calories a day to support your baby's growth. And this is a big time for growth! From fourteen to twenty-six weeks, your little one is further developing their central nervous system, eyes, ears, teeth, and external genitals. Your baby is also ramping up the development of their skeletal system and needs the necessary nutrients to form that. Your own digestive system might be running a little slower these days, so make sure you're consuming plenty of water to keep things moving!

SECOND-TRIMESTER FOODS

In addition to the nutrients you focused on in trimester one, you'll want to make sure you're getting enough of these too!

What It Is	What It Does	Where to Get It
Fiber	Promotes heart health, reduces the risk of preeclampsia, and aids in preventing constipation. Nobody wants to think about poop until you can't do it, but this trimester your hormones or growing baby might make it a little harder to go. Bonus: foods with fiber also have a variety of other healthy nutrients you and your baby need.	Red raspberries, peas, beans, lentils, avocado, artichokes, oatmeal
Protein	A crucial nutrient needed for baby's continued growth and the essential building block for human life. Babies grow quickly in the last few weeks of the second trimester especially, so it's very important that you incorporate a source of protein at every meal (and get it from a variety of both plant and animal sources).	Beans, lentils, tofu, chicken, turkey, beef, salmon (which also has DHA), eggs, and organ meats
Iron	Needed to make hemoglobin, a protein found in red blood cells that carries oxygen to tissues throughout the body. During pregnancy your iron needs almost *double* because you're making more blood to supply oxygen to your growing baby. Iron deficiency in pregnancy can cause fatigue, increase your risk of premature birth or low birth weight, and contribute to postpartum depression. Pregnant women need 27 mg of iron daily, as compared to 18 mg when you're not pregnant.	Chicken liver, bison, sardines, turkey, beef. Plant-based sources of iron, like dark leafy greens, beans, lentils, tofu, and cashews, are less bioavailable than animal sources, meaning they're not as easily absorbed by your body. Cooking in cast-iron pans can help fortify your food, and consuming these foods with a source of vitamin C can also help with absorption (think beef and broccoli or adding a squeeze of lemon to a spinach salad).

Vitamin D and calcium	These help build the baby's bones and teeth by working together to ensure healthy bone development. By week twenty, your baby's bones are visible on an ultrasound! Calcium also helps your circulatory, muscular, and nervous systems run properly, which is especially important during pregnancy. You need a minimum of 600 IU of vitamin D and 1,000 mg of calcium daily.	Get vitamin D from natural sunlight, salmon, and tuna. Calcium is found in dairy products like milk, yogurt, cheese, and cottage cheese, but for those avoiding dairy, you can get your calcium in edamame, spinach, and broccoli.

Mongolian Beef and Broccolini

Ingredients

- 1 cup jasmine rice
- 1 1/4 cup water
- 1 1/2 pounds pasture-raised flank steak
- 2 tablespoons avocado oil
- 6 garlic cloves, finely diced
- 1 tablespoon grated ginger
- 1/2 yellow bell pepper, thinly sliced
- 1/2 red bell pepper, thinly sliced
- 2 baby bok choy, trimmed and chopped
- 2 carrots, peeled and thinly sliced
- 2 handfuls broccolini, trimmed
- 2 green onions, roughly chopped
- 1 tablespoon sesame seeds for garnish

Sauce

- 1 tablespoon arrowroot starch
- 1 tablespoon water
- 1/3 cup coconut aminos
- 2 tablespoons tamari
- 1 tablespoon sesame oil

1 tablespoon rice vinegar

1 teaspoon honey

1. Get your rice started so it's done when the rest of your meal is. Combine rice and water in a saucepan and bring to a simmer. Once the rice is bubbling and foaming, turn the heat down and cover. Cook for 12 minutes. Turn off the burner and let your rice stand for 10 minutes before you "fluff" it with a spatula.
2. Slice your flank steak into thin, 2-inch pieces.
3. Heat the oil, garlic, and ginger in a large skillet on medium for 1 minute. Isn't this the best smell in the world? Yum.
4. Add in your steak and turn the heat to medium-high, cooking for 5 minutes.
5. It's veggie time! Add in your chopped peppers, bok choy, carrots, broccolini, and green onion, and cover. They'll need another 5 to 7 minutes to cook.
6. Meanwhile, whisk your arrowroot in a small bowl with 1 tablespoon water until dissolved. Add the coconut aminos, tamari, sesame oil, rice vinegar, and honey to make a slurry and add it into the skillet. Reduce the heat, stir, and let it cook for another few minutes.
7. Add a few more pieces of green onion and sesame seeds on top for garnish and serve over your rice.

Super Easy Lentil Bruschetta Salad

Ingredients

5 to 6 tomatoes, diced (vine-ripened is the best for this, but whatever you have access to works)

¼ small white onion, diced

1 cup basil, chopped

2 garlic cloves, minced

1 package precooked lentils (this is what makes it super easy!)

2 tablespoons extra-virgin olive oil

2 tablespoons balsamic vinegar

Salt and pepper to taste

¾ cup crumbled feta cheese (sub: 1 large avocado, diced)

1. Combine the chopped tomatoes, onion, basil, and garlic in a large mixing bowl.
2. Add in precooked lentils and mix well.
3. Dress with olive oil, balsamic vinegar, and salt and pepper to taste.
4. Add in feta cheese or avocado and gently combine.

PS: This is perfect on its own, on a bed of arugula or other greens, or as a dip with seed crackers or pita chips.

I will admit that I haven't always taken the best care of myself. I'm an emotional eater. I used to eat when I was super sad or would celebrate something good by eating. But the habits I built with Rebecca and Kristy truly changed the way I feel about myself and made nutrition and movement a key part of my self-care. The more I moved and paid attention to how I could nourish myself, the better I felt in my body.

These habits are so ingrained in me I don't even think about them that much anymore: they're as natural to me as brushing my teeth or tying my shoes (when I'm not wearing Crocs). Try not to compare yourself to anyone else. Just do your best to treat yourself and your body with love and kindness. You're amaaaaazing.

TEN

TWENTY WEEKS

Twenty weeks in, I couldn't believe my pregnancy was halfway through. My bump was finally bumping, my stretch marks were stretching, my skin was dry and weird, and even though I was still waking up with charley horses pretty much every night, Daryl still thought I was his dream woman.

At this point I still hadn't felt a kick yet. I knew I was pregnant from my bigger belly, but I would put a cheap heart monitor on my tummy almost every night to feel connected to my baby and to reassure myself that he was okay. The rhythm of your baby's heart beating inside you is the most beautiful sound you'll ever hear. I also splurged on a handheld ultrasound machine on Amazon. When I say *splurge* I mean I spent a thousand dollars on it, and everyone laughed at me and said I wasted the money, but to me, it wasn't a waste *at all*. I was anxious: I wasn't feeling kicks, and the doctor's office didn't do many ultrasounds, and seeing little hands and feet made me happy and reassured me that everything was fine. It was expensive, but that shit worked. So I win. Also, since it was during the COVID pandemic, this was the only way Daryl was allowed to see his son on the screen. So it was *definitely* worth it to see how happy it made him.

Around twenty-two weeks, I finally got my first real massage, specifically for pregnancy. (They have special ways to keep you comfortable and to position you safely.) There I was, relaxing, when I finally felt something move in my belly.

"I think he just kicked me!"

Then I felt it again, like Riley was saying, "Yep, that was me!"

I sat up and screamed for Daryl to come over and put his hands on my belly. He could feel our baby in there, too, and I teared up. *Wow,* I thought, *you really are in there.* It was the first time I felt pregnant. Kind of weird, since the kicking feels like an alien moving inside you, or like having what I call "bubble guts," when you eat something your tummy doesn't agree with and it starts to push a giant fart down. It's bizarre, and I loved it.

Once the kicking started, I knew this was legit and that I needed to get a nursery ready. My house at the time had only one extra bedroom because, as I've mentioned, we live with my two adult brothers. The only other bedroom available for my boy was in between both of my brothers' rooms . . . on the opposite side of our house, farthest from our bedroom.

I don't recommend this at all, but we started the process of moving into a new house. During a pandemic. While I was pregnant AF. I knew we needed the baby close to us and that our current bedroom wasn't going to work as a nursery. So while the new house got ready for us, I got ready for baby. You know what I mean: mama started shopping. Baby stuff is *expensive,* but Target and Amazon have everything you need; your baby will love you whether you have the fanciest things or hand-me-downs, and half the stuff I bought I never even used (shout-out to the full newborn wardrobe we bought at Target, only to have him in zip-up pajamas for the first three months of his life, and the Frida Mom kit I bought to take care of my vag, only to have a C-section). It feels really good to nest and buy things, but it's hard to know what you're going to need until you actually have the baby.

Being pregnant during the worst of the COVID pandemic (we hope) meant that Daryl and I had a lot of time together during this pregnancy. Any other time in my career, I'd have been on the go, traveling around the world for shows and appearances. I look back on this time as a special season for us: we were in our own little bubble, sleeping on the couch, going for hikes, and ordering our meals in. We were super privileged to have all our needs met, to not be worried about losing our house or our jobs, and to have access to the health care that I needed, even if it meant that I went to every appointment alone. In the grand scheme of things, that's just a small thing, but it always made me think about the women who go through this experience on their own without a partner waiting for them at home: y'all are amazing, you're heroes, you're queens. And for all the other mamas who went through a pandemic pregnancy and didn't get to hold your partner's hand during an ultrasound, or who heard the results of a blood test alone, I feel you, and you are brave. If you had to hear bad news when you were all alone in a little room, my heart breaks for you, and I'm hugging you so hard right now.

Anywhere between eighteen and twenty-four weeks, you might get an additional ultrasound to check how baby is developing and to screen for fetal abnormalities. I knew from the jump I'd want to get as many ultrasounds as possible, but when I heard there was a 3D ultrasound, I knew I had to have one. But *then* I saw a celebrity I knew post about getting a 3D ultrasound at home. That changed the whole game for me. I had no idea that was a possibility—a doctor could come to your house? Daryl could be there? My *family* could be there? I'm going to say right now that we paid a shit-ton of money for this, and I know that it's out of reach for most people. But this is the reality of my life, and I want to keep it *fully* real with you: I got to write a fat check and have a doctor bring a whole-ass ultrasound machine into our living room to watch my favorite show of all time: my baby.

> ## TREAT YOURSELF
>
> Obviously not everyone can have a doctor come to their *house* and give them a special ultrasound. But I also think that doing something a little extra during your pregnancy is well deserved. If you want to sneak a peek at your baby, there are 3D ultrasounds at some malls and shopping centers. Or just go get yourself a massage! You deserve it.

My family is really close (I mean, again, my adult brothers live with me), and I knew that whether we got great news or horrible news, I wanted them there with me. So we all crowded onto the same couch that I slept on: me, Daryl, my parents, my brothers, my managers, my uncle . . . the whole Trainor Team showed up to see our baby in 3D. Everyone knew that it wasn't just for fun but that the doctor would be checking to make sure the baby's brain, spine, and organs were developing correctly, and that they could be here for good news or life-changing bad news. We were still laughing and joking—that's what we do—but I could tell that everyone was a little tense too. A 3D ultrasound isn't like going to see a 3D movie—you don't need special glasses, nothing pops out of the screen—but once they squeeze the goo on your tummy and start moving that wand around, you see your baby for real. The last time we'd had an ultrasound, he looked like a little ghostly white blob. But this time we could see his face: his cute little nose, his sweet mouth. He looked like a little doll, and while everyone oohed and aahed over this perfect little boy, I had my breath held and my eyes locked on the doctor. *Did he just squint? Flinch? Is something wrong? Is he sweaty?* This poor guy couldn't have a private thought or a normal facial expression without me thinking something was horribly wrong.

I was about to burst and knew I couldn't hold it in any longer. I looked at the doctor and said, "Is he okay?"

He looked at me and said, "He's perfect."

Joy and relief swept through my whole body. My mom's hand squeezed mine, and Daryl pulled me in for a kiss. Our baby was *perfect*.

"Can you just make sure it's really a boy?" I asked, because, you know, *people are wrong sometimes!* Everyone laughed, but the doctor for real checked. Suddenly my entire family and team were looking at my baby's balls. Guess I couldn't argue with that. Yep, still a boy.

This day is one of my very favorite memories: everyone I loved in one room, pouring all their love into this little baby. I don't know how long this procedure would be in the doctor's office, but I know that we had almost two hours of time to peek into the little universe inside me. I knew we were seeing the inside of my body, but it just seemed too incredible to be true. Right here, right *inside me*, there was this perfect little baby boy swallowing and sucking his thumb while I watched TV or wrote music or went for a walk. I couldn't stop smiling the entire time, thinking about what it would be like to see him in my arms. The doctor took pictures for us to keep, and I told him, "All right man, no pressure, but you're gonna get the announcement pic, so focus and make it a good one." He nailed it.

ELEVEN

I FAILED

The first time I thought about gestational diabetes, it was at the sixteen-week appointment. COVID was still raging, and Daryl still couldn't come to appointments with me, which was always a bummer, but switching doctors made me look forward to my time with Dr. Solky. We'd gone over my family history, and my mom had mentioned *something* about gestational diabetes, but I couldn't remember what specifically. Something about drinking too much orange juice?

The test was straight-up gnarly: I had to fast for eight or more hours beforehand and then drink a bottle of what tasted like cough syrup. It's famously nasty; the nurse even told me, "If you throw up, just let us know." I didn't throw up, but I chugged it as fast as I could and waited for the results. I passed, and I drove home feeling like a queen. I was healthy, the baby was healthy, and nothing else mattered.

The next check for gestational diabetes was at twenty-four weeks, and I was prepared. I'd spent a lot of time on YouTube looking up what it meant to have gestational diabetes, and I was fully freaked out: it looked like a full-time job to manage your blood sugar, and I was worried about any potential risks to the baby. These women had sad, boring meal plans and had to constantly go on walks and test their blood sugar. Couldn't be me. I was eating pretty well, exercising, and ready to ace this test again.

WHAT IS GESTATIONAL DIABETES?

Gestational diabetes affects between 2 to 5 percent of pregnant women and is a (usually) temporary condition where your body does not produce enough insulin to regulate your blood sugar. According to the American Pregnancy Association, risk factors include

- being overweight or obese
- a lack of physical activity
- previous gestational diabetes or prediabetes
- polycystic ovary syndrome
- diabetes in an immediate family member
- previously delivering a baby weighing more than nine pounds
- race—women who are Black, Hispanic, American Indian, and Asian American have a higher risk of developing gestational diabetes[1]

I decided to fully cut out carbs and sugar for the weeks leading up to the second test, and I felt confident as I chugged down that gross glucose drink that I would pass with flying colors. I wouldn't get the results until the next day, but again, I drove home feeling like I was on top of the world. And I was, until the next morning. Daryl woke me up on the couch. The moment I opened my eyes, I knew it was bad, because he *always* let me sleep in.

"Babe," he said, "I'm so sorry. You have gestational diabetes and you have to go to the doctor."

"Are you serious?" I truly thought I was still in a dream . . . a nightmare.

He was serious. He told me over and over it was going to be okay, but the first words to cross my mind were *I failed*. It felt like my heart fell through the floor. I called my doctor, crying, confessing that I had actually had a Pop-Tart recently. She assured me that it was not the Pop-Tart, that it was my genetics, and that my baby and I would be okay. But it didn't feel okay. It didn't feel like I'd failed a blood test; it felt like I was failing at pregnancy. I know it sounds dramatic, but if you've gone through this, you know exactly how scary it is. I suddenly had a whole new job on top of my other full-time jobs: I was literally dieting, plus testing my blood sugar four times a day every day (pricking my finger, dabbing the blood on a tiny strip, and putting it into a machine). Every time I did it I was holding my breath, hoping that my blood sugar wasn't too high. I had to think about every single bite of food I put into my mouth and what it would do to my blood sugar, and y'all know I was already anxious as hell—I bought my own ultrasound machine!

CAN I PREVENT GESTATIONAL DIABETES?

There aren't any guarantees, but healthy habits go a long way. According to the American Pregnancy Association, eating healthy, staying active, keeping your pregnancy weight gain in control, and starting pregnancy at a healthy weight can lower your risk.[2] Aside from that last one, I did all that! But it's also a genetic thing, so it made sense that I had it since my mom had it and my grandma had it.

I could afford the machine and the needles and the testing strips and the alcohol wipes, but this stuff is expensive, and that's a whole other added stress level for a mama. Every time I had to go to the pharmacy to get another sixty-dollar or eighty-dollar box of testing strips, I'd think about how heavy that cost would be for some people, especially people who have to do this for their entire *lives*. It's not just the cost of the supplies—it's the time it takes to learn about what's happening to your body and how to manage it, and the time it takes to make sure you're eating properly and keeping track of everything you're eating. Your time is also money, and not everyone has the time to spend counting every bite of food that passes their lips. When I posted a TikTok about my gestational diabetes, I got tons of comments from people around the world who do this shit every day forever, and from kids in the hospital due to diabetes. It was a huge perspective shift: my suffering was small and temporary. This would be my focus until the baby was born—*when it often just mysteriously disappears?*—and if some people could do this forever, I could do it for a few months.

But it sucked. The information I got (not from Kristy!) was confusing, and I had to fill out a spreadsheet for a dietitian recording everything I ate and what my blood sugar results were after eating. I was paranoid that everything I ate would spike my blood sugar and hurt the baby, and I avoided carbs entirely. I unintentionally put myself on a keto diet and felt sick and run-down. I was doing everything I was told and was still informed we might have to consider insulin to control my blood sugar. I was going nuts.

Being the sweetest husband that he is, Daryl secretly asked my dietitian whether it was okay to have pizza on my birthday. She said yes, as long as we did it early in the evening and went for a walk after. When he told me the surprise, I cried—not happy tears at first, because I was so terrified and didn't want to do it. He called her on the phone in front of me to prove to me that it was safe. Pizza is my favorite food, and I barely enjoyed it because I was so worried about what it would do to my blood sugar. I had three slices of the thinnest thin crust available and took that walk right after . . . and it was *fine*. But I still spent Christmas watching everyone have a beautiful meal while I ate a sad little caprese salad.

When people ask, "How's the pregnancy going?" they're not expecting you to say, "Well, actually, I have gestational diabetes." But that's exactly what I did to Ryan Seacrest when I was doing promo for the Christmas album. I wasn't planning to bring it up, but he asked how it was going, and the truth was that I spent most of my days freaking out about my blood sugar! Poor guy, he looked panicked and asked whether I was going to be okay. I knew deep down I would be, but it was lonely and overwhelming, and I wanted any other mama who was watching and going through the same thing to know that she wasn't alone. I was here, too, pricking my finger and going on my little walks, paranoid and worried I would spike my blood sugars.

As shitty as this experience was, I've also never had a great relationship with food. I'm the "All About That Bass" girl. I've never been a size two, and I'm not trying to be, but my experience with gestational diabetes was also the first time I really paid attention to how I ate and how it affected me. Once I actually started working with Kristy—bless her—I knew that how I nourished myself wasn't just about losing pregnancy weight; this was about my life and the kind of life I want to have with my family, my future kids. I don't want to be stuck in a loop where I eat my feelings and feel horrible physically and emotionally. I don't want to binge-eat until I'm curled up on the couch in pain, moaning about how I fucked up. I don't want to feel shitty and tired and have acne and be getting sick all the time. I don't want to feel stressed or shamed about what I eat or don't eat. So many of my physical and emotional struggles are linked with my relationship with food, and finally, at twenty-eight, I can say that I'm in a place I never saw for myself.

I'm thirty pounds lighter than I was *before* I got pregnant, but that's not the biggest change: I can't remember the last time I had a zit or got sick. I went from 220 pounds at my most pregnant to 155. Remember, when I first got pregnant, I was 185 pounds. I used to be a Sleeping Beauty who would wake up around noon, and now I wake up every morning by six thirty with my husband and my baby. Who the fuck am I? Someone I've always wanted to be and never thought I could be.

Bestie, what I'm saying is that food is crucial in all aspects of life, *especially pregnancy*. When I stopped using it as a crutch for my emotions, it started to become a tool. What you're doing right now is the most important, sacred work your body has ever done. *Food is fuel*. But I still enjoy my pizza every other week with a giant salad to start so I don't go in starving. See, I'm a new woman!

The best thing I learned from Kristy is to *listen* to my body. Be *mindful* of my body. Am I hungry or am I bored? Are my poops normal? Did that meal just make my stomach hurt? It's amazing how in tune you can actually be with your body. You and your baby deserve to be nourished and taken care of, to grow happy and healthy together. It took more than just a few months of working with Kristy and my therapist, but it was *worth it*, and so are you, for real.

TWELVE

SECOND-TRIMESTER CHECKLIST

Being pregnant during COVID was absolutely bizarre. There was so much I didn't get to do and so much I didn't *have* to do. Not being able to gather with people indoors got me out of a few of my worst nightmares: namely, a baby shower and a gender reveal. I love my friends and family, but I am also a straight-up control freak and I would not be able to sit through an event where people gave me presents that I might not even want. I know, I know, I'm a freak for this. But am I? Because I personally think it's very normal to want to decide what exactly you want in your home. Anyway, your second trimester might be when your loved ones want to get together and throw you a baby shower, and it's when you're officially closer to the end of your pregnancy than the beginning of it. In other words, shit's getting real.

SET UP YOUR REGISTRY

This is (or can be) so fun, and also overwhelming. Before you go ham and decide you need to be signed up for every possible baby product under the sun, get off Instagram and look around your house. Do you really have room for that giant baby swing? Do you have a chair that can work for nursing, or do you absolutely need a rocker? I'm saying this as a girl who kept the Amazon delivery drivers *busy* and who also bought (and registered for) a ton of stuff that ended up being donated without ever being opened. If you can get out of your house and actually go *see* things, do it, and do it with your partner. It's their baby, too, and they might have some good ideas (or at least some funny ones that you can laugh at later).

TRAVEL

Again, LOL, we did not get to do this, and I really wasn't all that disappointed. I travel a lot for work, and being forced to stay home was ultimately really good for me. But if traveling is your thing, now's the time to do it. The guidelines change based on your pregnancy, your provider, and the airline, but trust: you're not going to want to sit on a plane when your belly is the size of a beach ball. I know lots of new parents who treated themselves to a babymoon as a last hurrah before their baby arrived, but you don't need to take some big, flashy trip. Maybe you want to spend some time with family who live out of town, and maybe the two of you just want to book a night at a hotel for a staycation. If this is your thing, now's the time to do it.

EXPLORE YOUR CHILDCARE OPTIONS

I don't know how many rants I can fit in this book, but here's another: the cost of childcare went up 41 percent during the pandemic, and now some families spend up to 20 percent of their income on childcare.[1] You know, because parenting wasn't stressful enough. There are some cities where you need to be on a waitlist for certain childcare providers before you're even pregnant, in which case this advice is already too late for you, sorry. Hopefully you and your partner have already talked about your budget and about what you want for your family: maybe one of you is going to stay home and handle childcare duties while the other works (shout-out to Daryl for this!), and maybe you're both heading back to work and you'll need a childcare center or a nanny. Whatever you do, spend time getting referrals, reading reviews, and going *in person* to see the place and meet the people that might be taking care of your most important person.

TAKE PHOTOS

Of course we were taking pictures the entire pregnancy, but I waited until the very end of my second trimester to do a real shoot, because I really wanted that bump-bump. Whatever you decide to do, make sure you're documenting this special time in your life.

DO ALL THE THINGS

Okay, not *all* the things, but this is the trimester where your energy will be up and you'll be feeling good. Before you go into nesting-and-resting mode, do what you're up for doing.

MEET TEAM MAMA

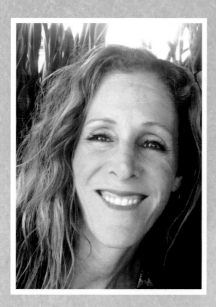

Dr. Karyn Solky,
ob-gyn

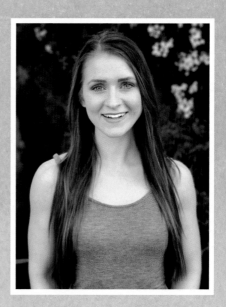

Rebecca Stanton,
my personal trainer

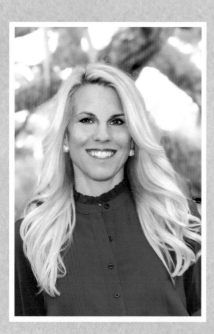

Kristy Morrell,
registered dietitian

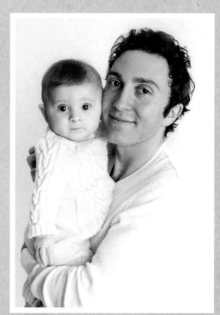

Chaya Tenenbaum   http://www.cgphotographyla.com

My husband, Daryl,
aka "Spy Kids"

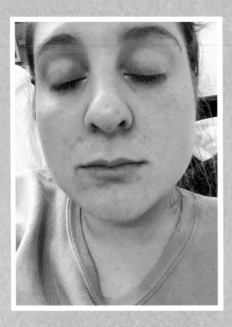

My perioral dermatitis flaring up and being itchy AF.

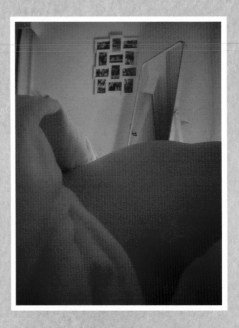

First evidence of a bump!

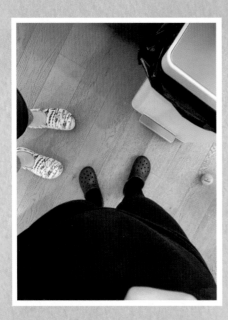

More evidence of a bump!

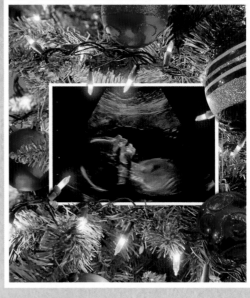

Our holiday-themed pregnancy announcement pic!

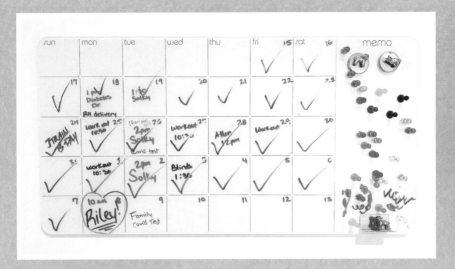

The final countdown calendar.

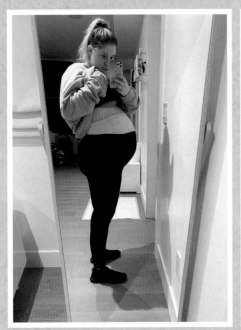

How is there not a toddler in there?! Final bump pic.

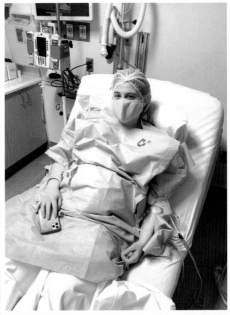

Moments before my C-section, freaking the fuck out but also so excited!

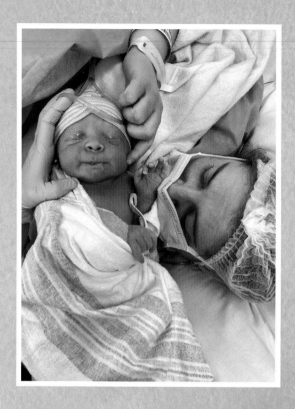

Touching
him to make
sure he's real.

Finally—first time
getting to hold
my baby boy!

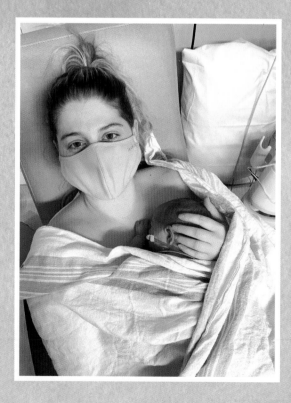

I thought my
ankles were
going to explode
like grenades.

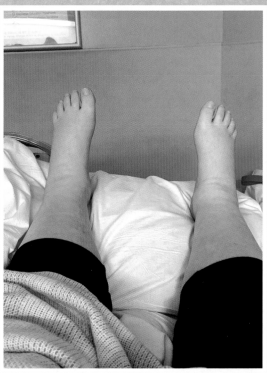

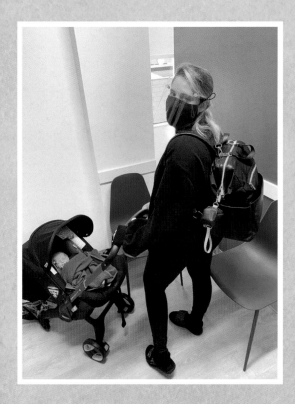

Feeling like a
boss mom at the
pediatrician's
office, though I
could barely walk.

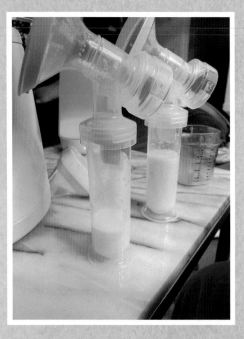

The most milk I ever got.
Proof of how much bigger my
right boob is than my left.

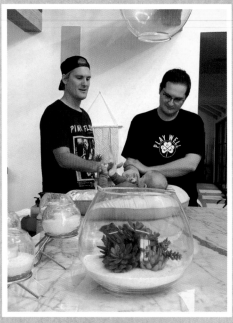

I caught my brothers trying
to hang out with Riley.

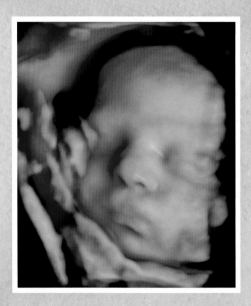

The final ultrasound
of Riley. This was my
background on my phone
for so long. It's crazy how
accurate these are.

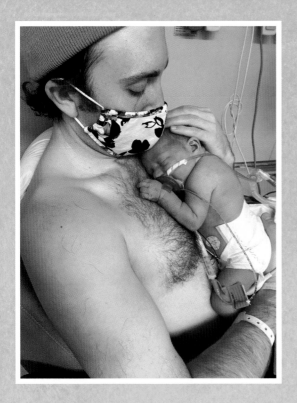

Daryl getting his skin-to-skin time.

When I met Riley for the first time. I couldn't stop petting him.

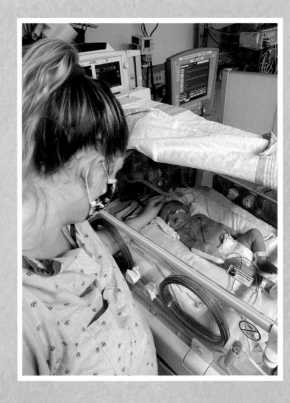

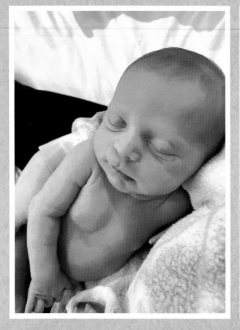

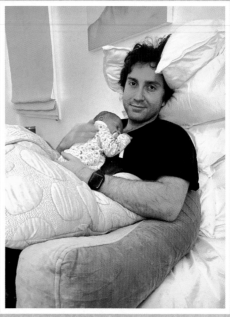

My gorgeous C-section baby. He even came out with a tan. Ha ha.

An example of how beautiful but exhausting these months were.

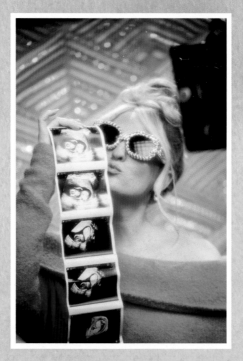

Pregnancy #2 is already completely different. Can't wait to tell you all about it!

PART THREE

TRIMESTER THREE

THIRTEEN

YOU'RE ALMOST THERE

It's the home stretch! *You're so motherfuckin' close.*

This trimester is all about nesting, resting, and anticipating the arrival of your sweet little baby. It's also when I fully gave up on hair, makeup, and any of the cute maternity outfits I bought before I even had a bump. My boobs were huge, my belly felt enormous, and my personal style became "this fits and is loose." My belly was so big it felt like I couldn't control my body. The number of times I walked into walls or swung the refrigerator door into my belly because of the size of me was embarrassing and straight-up dangerous. I don't know whether this was a pregnancy symptom or I was just massive and delirious, but I've never been clumsier in my life. Like, it was my job to spill large glasses of ice water. I was a mess. I lived in Daryl's sweatshirts and pajama pants and the one pair of leggings that still fit. I didn't even recognize my reflection, and I'm not just being dramatic. I'd pass by a mirror and think, "OMG, who's that? Is she okay?"

She was not okay. I'm being dramatic, but the biggest lie anyone told me about the third trimester was that I'd be "a little uncomfortable." No, I was hella uncomfortable and straight up in pain. Everything hurt: I used to cry about not being able to feel any kicks, and now this baby was doing full-on karate inside me, and I swear his little feet were about to break through my ribs. People would say, "You'll miss it someday!" And I'd say, "Hell no, I won't!" I discovered what my sciatic nerve was when I felt pain zipping like lightning from my lower back down my legs. Bending down hurt so bad I couldn't pull my own pants up or get off the toilet without help. Every bump in the car made it feel like my stomach was going to explode or the baby was going to fall out of my vagina. Guys, the bottoms of my feet hurt *even when I wasn't walking.* They hurt so much that I'd sit in the shower just to get off my feet and wonder out loud how people actually walked all day, as if I hadn't been one of those people for most of my life. If I *had* to stand, I'd fantasize about going back to bed. If you'd told me that my baby was three feet tall and weighed sixty pounds, I would have believed you, because that's what it felt like I was carrying around all day. I was certain he was already a toddler in there. That bump that I'd been dreaming of was so big that Daryl had to shave my legs for me. TBH that's no big deal for him, but I missed being able to move around without my body aching. As excited as I was to finally meet our baby, I had a lot on my mind too.

LET'S TALK ABOUT LEAVE

As you know, I don't have a regular job with a steady paycheck and regular hours. I'm in no way complaining—I'm lucky AF and I love absolutely everything about what I do—but there's no set maternity leave policy for an entertainer. If I don't work, I don't get paid, and I really wanted to take time off *before* the baby arrived so I could try to enjoy the experience as much as possible and keep my stress levels down. But the timing worked out for me perfectly, and my team is amazing. The Christmas album dropped in September (bizarre, but that's how it's done), and I had already done all the work I had to do other than promote and post about it. I was still testing my blood sugar multiple times a day and sleeping on the couch, and we were still doing construction on a house that was about halfway finished, but December 17 was my first day of maternity leave. By January 1 I was free to just enjoy my last weeks of pregnancy.

Again, I know how lucky I am. While I was writing this book, I was in a magazine office for an interview about my song "Bad for Me," and there was a pregnant employee lying on a couch looking like she was about to pop. I don't usually do this, but she was basically crowning, and I barked, "You should be home! You shouldn't have to work!" I did this right in front of her bosses, which was probably not cool. But for real, she should have time off and not be worried about "wasting" her maternity leave before the baby arrives. My mom reminded me that she worked in the jewelry store she and my dad owned *until the day she gave birth*. She spent all day on her feet until she delivered the baby. It breaks my heart that women don't get the leave and the rest they deserve during this time. Rant over.

As special as it was to have this time together as a couple before we welcomed our first child, I was also really scared to take this time off. Entertainment is an industry where if you're booked and busy, you're blessed, and saying no to work can be risky. I'd worked with my team and everyone agreed with my leave and supported me, but there was still that voice inside me telling me *Maybe you should be working right now*. I'm lucky to have a team and a career that made it possible for me to take *any* time off: maternity leave in the United States is absolute garbage, and a lot of you know that firsthand. But beyond the *ability* to take time for you and your baby, there's also *what you want*. I'm a woman who wants it all: I want my career, I want a bunch of kids, I want time with my friends and family, I want to have my cake and give everyone else a slice too. I wanted to take that time off, but I also wanted to be writing music and performing.

I was raised by parents who owned their own small business. I grew up seeing my mom as the ultimate mom *and* as a boss. Being a small-business owner meant she had the flexibility to get me and my brothers to school and take us to all our activities, but being the boss also meant that sometimes, work *did* have to come first. I never held it against her or resented it, and I always assumed that when I became a mom, I'd be like her: I'd do it all, and I'd do it with a smile. But living it—even before the baby arrived—felt different. This was a new kind of pressure; it wouldn't just be my team relying on me, it would be my *child*. What would it look like to balance these parts of my life? When would I be able to get back to work after he arrived . . . and would I want to? Any therapist out there will tell you to stay in the moment and stop projecting, but I couldn't help it: the closer we got to our due date, the closer I got to the end of my leave.

THE BIRTH PLAN

When a nurse asked, "Do you have a birth plan?" I was confused. "Uh, don't *you* make the plan? Am I supposed to have one?? Am I terrible that I don't?" Apparently, women can make literal birth plans with all the kinds of details they'd like to incorporate, like a vision board for childbirth. I get wanting to make a plan—I love a plan!—but one of the wisest things that Dr. Solky told me was that childbirth doesn't really care about your plans. The only plan I could think of was to have a healthy baby. I (obviously) didn't make a birth plan, but other mamas I know did, and they suggested you talk through the following with your partner and your provider:

- Who do you want in the room? Just your partner? Your parents? A videographer? Obviously with COVID I was not going to be rolling in with my whole fam, but if there are people you do—or don't!—want in the room, get on the same page with your partner. Apparently, when my mom was in labor, my dad would just roll into the room with random guests: their employees, friends, distant relatives . . . people my mom straight up didn't like. My parents *were* aligned on lying to my dad's mom about the due date so she wouldn't show up, but I guess my mom could have used a birth plan, because my dad thought birth was a party.

- What kind of labor do you want? If you *could* have it go to plan, would you want an epidural or a birth without painkillers? Do you want to have a water birth?
- What do you want to have happen right after birth? Do you want your partner to cut the cord, or your niece who snuck into the room (LOL)? I knew—even if I didn't write a plan—that I wanted skin-to-skin contact with my baby before they did all the newborn stuff.

COVID made it hard to have much of a plan. By the end of my pregnancy, Daryl could be in the hallway outside the waiting room during my appointments, but we knew that I wouldn't be able to have my mom in the delivery room with us like I'd always assumed she'd be.

Good thing I didn't have a birth plan, because Riley was straight-up trolling me. At my thirty-week appointment, he was *perfect*. I'm talking head down, ready to go. I couldn't believe it. He was in position? My boy!

Two weeks later, my friend who is a doula asked me, "Do you feel him dropping so low like he's falling out of you?" I was so confused because I didn't feel that at all. At thirty-two weeks, this kid was *sideways* inside me. No wonder it felt like he was going to bust through my rib cage; I could see his little feet pressing through my belly. "That's not the exit!" I'd say to him every time he kicked my ribs. I was worried: if he was breech, I'd have to get a C-section, and I really wanted to push a baby out. Dr. Solky told me not to worry, Riley had plenty of time to get into position; and at the thirty-four-week appointment, he had finally figured it out. His head was in the perfect position, his feet were no longer stuck to my ribs, and I was *excited.*

"Do you think I'll be able to push him out?" I asked Dr. Solky.

"Looks like it!" she replied, and I rushed out to the lobby to tell Daryl the good news.

Riley, though, had other plans. By the thirty-six-week sonogram, he was back to his old tricks and fully breech. I'd already started watching YouTube videos about labor and delivery, and I was worried. Would he have time to get into position? He was *just there!* How'd he get this turned around?

I saw Dr. Solky a few days later to see whether Riley had figured it out, and it had gotten worse. He was somehow in a jackknife position: his butt was down, his head was in my left ribs, and his feet were in my right ribs. Now that he's a year old and just got glasses I can joke that he just got lost in there, but I was *scared.* Dr. Solky explained that it was unlikely Riley would get into the right position in time and that we should plan for a C-section. I was devastated and terrified. I had spent weeks watching labor videos and imagining my water breaking spontaneously like in the movies, and now I was planning for a major surgery. I cried as soon as I saw Daryl in the waiting room. I'd never broken a bone or even had stitches before, and it's not like I thought vaginal birth was going to be painless, but a C-section is *intense.* When I was still on the car ride home, the hospital called to schedule the C-section, or as the lady on the phone put it, "What day would you like your son to be born?" I was picking our son's birthday! I took the first available date they offered, February 8. It would be the first day of my thirty-ninth week of pregnancy.

Then I went home and did exactly what you thought I'd do: I watched a ton of YouTube videos about C-sections and freaked myself out. I'll spare you the details, except for the video where a woman went off about how having a C-section "doesn't count" as giving birth. She's wrong, and so is anyone who tells you anything like that. Having a baby—however you do it—is amazing, and so are you. Baby coming out of you equals birth.

But I was still holding out hope that Riley would figure it out. When I posted on Instagram about the baby being breech, I got tons of messages from followers and from celebrities filled with advice to get him turned around. I did all of it: cat-cow stretches, downward dogs, hanging upside-down off the couch—it didn't work, and it just freaked me out more. Riley wasn't turning around, and he was going to enter this world on February 8.

A birth plan is *just* a plan, a best-case scenario for how you'd like your birth experience to go. I'm grateful that we didn't have one, because when it became clear that this birth was not going to meet *any* of my expectations, I had a big, beautiful revelation. To *surrender.* Surrender my body, surrender to what needed to be done. I knew I didn't have control, and I didn't want it. I just wanted my baby out of me safely. Even if it meant a C-section. My stylist and good friend told me how she had two C-sections and to think of them as a spa day. You walk into the hospital (your hotel) with no labor pains, get your baby out in under ten minutes, and have nurses tend to you for three days.

FOURTEEN

THIRD-TRIMESTER CHECKLIST

If you've already bought more baby clothes than your baby could possibly wear (guilty), take a break from shopping and take care of these details.

DOUBLE-CHECK YOUR MATERNITY LEAVE POLICY AT WORK

Do you have a plan for when your last day of work is? Are you covered by short-term disability? Take the time to make sure all your paperwork is in place with human resources, and check with your manager to make sure everyone is clear on a coverage plan for while you're out and that everyone is aware of the first and last dates of your leave.

TOUR THE HOSPITAL OR BIRTH CENTER

Assuming there's not a pandemic, you can typically go take a tour to familiarize yourself with the parking situation and the check-in process and even see the rooms where you could give birth.

PICK YOUR PEDIATRICIAN

I totally forgot to do this, and luckily Dr. Solky came through with the best recommendation, Dr. Scott Cohen. (His book, *Eat, Sleep, Poop*, was the most helpful thing we read.) Your ob-gyn may have some suggestions, but check with your insurance to see who is in-network and how you can establish that care relationship for your baby.

BABY-PROOF THE HOUSE

They're not going to be crawling around for a while, but there are things you can do to make your home safer, even for a newborn:

- Make sure you have carbon monoxide and smoke detectors.
- Move the crib away from any heaters, wall decorations, windows, or lamps.
- Put a thick rug or pad beneath the changing table.

WASH THE BABY CLOTHES YOU BOUGHT

Remove the tags and run them through the machine with gentle, baby-friendly detergent.

INSTALL YOUR CAR SEAT

Newborns need rear-facing seats, and they need to be installed correctly. There are a billion YouTube videos to show you how, but many cities also have programs where you can have them installed or checked for free.

PREP YOUR MEALS

Having some healthy, easy meals stashed away in your freezer will take cooking off your to-do list when the baby arrives. Everyone always offers to drop off dinner, but you can freeze waffles, pancakes, and breakfast burritos (anything you can eat with one hand is great). And if anyone asks what you need for the baby, give them a specific meal to drop off!

THE NAME GAME

I've heard lots of parents say they couldn't name their baby until they laid eyes on them. I admire that restraint, because I picked out our baby's name the first month of pregnancy. Daryl and I had a few rules: the name had to be gender neutral, and it couldn't be the name of anyone we knew. Daryl liked *Parker* (as in Peter Parker), but I had my heart set on *Riley* right away. Riley it was, boy or girl. Here's my one piece of advice for names: don't tell anyone the name unless you're sure they won't be a jerk about it. People are super judgmental about baby names and love to give their opinions, whether or not you ask for it. It's obnoxious, honestly.

My family loved the name Riley so much that my mom gave me a mountain of personalized gifts that Christmas: blankets, onesies, a sick LED light. One problem: I'd decided a few weeks before that I loved the name Brody, and I hadn't told her. My brothers and Daryl were cracking up every time I opened another gift that said *Riley*. In the end, I (obviously) changed my mind again, but I bet baby Brody wouldn't have cared if he'd been wrapped in a Riley swaddle.

If you're struggling to unite on a name, you can go to the Social Security website and search the most popular names from any year. It's kind of cool to see what names were trending five, ten, or one hundred years ago.[1]

A WORD ON ADVICE

People. Love. To. Give. Pregnant. Women. Advice. They love it! I swear there are people who are just hiding in the shadows waiting for a pregnant woman to walk by so they can jump out, rub her belly, and tell her five things she's doing wrong. TBH, one benefit of a COVID pregnancy was that I didn't have a lot of face time with strangers. But don't worry, they still slid into my DMs! I have a little mom group filled with mamas who all have babies around Riley's age, and I fired up the group chat and asked them for the best advice they got during their pregnancy. Keep in mind, the best advice is the kind you *ask* for . . . so take even these with a grain of salt.

Before having your first baby is likely the last time in your life that you can be wholeheartedly carefree and selfish. When that kiddo comes, from that day on, the center of your world shifts and the weight of worry about them is at the forefront *all the time*. Take your pregnant months to truly care for yourself. If you want to binge TV, do it. If you want to leisurely stroll every aisle at the grocery store, do it. If you want to take naps on your days off . . . definitely do it!

I wish I'd thought of my first pregnancy this way. Next time, I'll have Riley along for the ride and everything will be different!

All of this is temporary, just a brief period of your life. However it feels is not forever. Ride those waves—exhaustion, fear, anxiety, joy—and know that another wave is coming.

This is amazing advice. Ride the waves, mama.

Speak up for yourself and your baby. A good doctor will listen to you and hear your concerns.

I didn't write that one, I promise, but I obviously fully endorse it!

Nobody tells you that with a C-section, you might not experience an immediate, movie-like obsession with your just-birthed child. If you're wondering how long you'll search for the connection everyone else seemingly has on day one, the answer is only: not forever. C-sections are not the easy way out, and the usual meds recommended for pain management postdelivery can roll in with a darkness that renders you static. I needed the medication for pain management, but what I also needed was for someone to tell me that the fog would clear and I would love my baby—in that movie-like way—once I was through it. The whole of myself simply just had to catch up to the blunt and abrupt transition of baby-outside-body. So to the mom warrioring through C-section recovery and wondering if all her bonding attempts will ever take: the fog will clear. I repeat: the fog will clear.

Amen.

FIFTEEN

THIRD-TRIMESTER FOOD AND FITNESS

Keep It Moving with Rebecca

The goal this trimester is just to keep moving. By this point, you're bigger, you might be uncomfortable, and it's not as easy to get up off the floor. So again, the goal this trimester is simply to keep moving, even if it's just a walk around the block or a few squats. Do what you can and what feels good!

Equipment Needed:

Dumbbells (5-to-8-pound weights or whatever you feel comfortable with)

Stability ball

Chair

Exercise mat

Glute band

Your Affirmation:

I'm strong. I'm capable. I'm ready.

Third-Trimester Fitness

SET 1

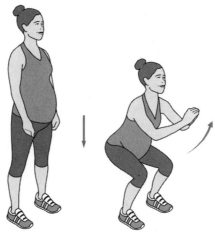

Deep Squat Stretch

Yes, even though it's a stretch, this will be part of your workout during your third trimester! Spread your feet out so they are a little wider than shoulder-width apart and your toes are rotated out. Lower yourself into a deep squat stretch. Hold this position for 20 to 30 seconds.

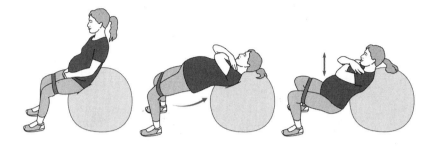

Banded Glute Bridge on Stability Ball

Step into the glute band and raise it until it fits snugly around your thighs. Slowly and carefully sit on the stability ball and roll out until your back is flat and your shins are at a 90-degree angle with your upper back on the stability ball. Lower your booty toward the ground while pressing your knees against the band the whole time. Bring your hips back up to the starting position. Repeat for additional reps.

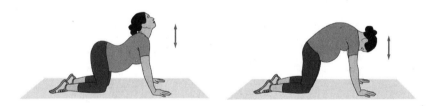

Cat-Cow Stretch

Start in a tabletop position with your hands and knees shoulder-width apart on the floor. Inhale deeply while curving your lower back: bring your head up, looking at the sky, and point your tailbone up too. Then exhale and bring your tummy/abdomen in, arching your back and bringing your head and tailbone down like a cat does when it stretches.

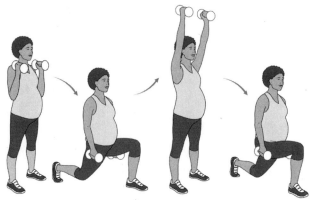

Alternating Hammer Press Lunge

Stand with your feet shoulder-width apart, both dumbbells by your shoulders. Step back into a reverse lunge position and step back in. As you step back in, hammer press the dumbbells overhead. Repeat on the other side by stepping back with the opposite leg and stepping back into a hammer press. Repeat and alternate legs as you go.

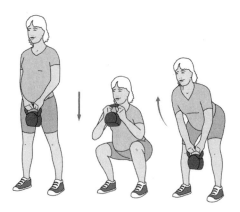

Squat to Deadlift

Start with your feet shoulder-width apart, holding a dumbbell with both hands so that it hangs in front of you between your legs, toes slightly rotated out. Squat down until your hips reach a 90-degree angle, then stand up and hinge forward into a deadlift position, making sure your back is straight the entire time. Stand back up straight and start again with the squat, alternating from the squat to the deadlift.

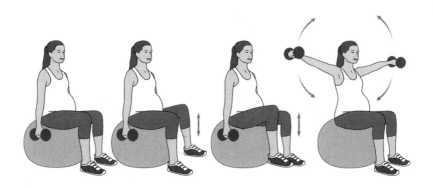

Stability Ball March with Dumbbell Lateral Raise

Start seated on the stability ball with the dumbbells by your sides. March by alternating leg lifts, one at a time. After each set of marches, raise the dumbbells laterally with your arms straight until your wrists are even with your shoulders. Lower your dumbbells back down and repeat for additional reps.

Let's Eat with Kristy

You've almost made it! You're probably feeling pretty tired, and that's totally normal. The size and the way that your baby is positioned can make sleeping difficult. Try to get rest when you can, and be gentle with yourself. In these final weeks, continue to pay attention to all the good nutrients you've focused on throughout the pregnancy, and make sure you're getting enough of these:

What It Is	What It Does	Where to Get It
Vitamin K	Helps your blood to clot and is essential in preventing serious bleeding during childbirth. It is also important to help maintain healthy bones in both you *and* your baby.	Leafy green vegetables like spinach, arugula, kale, turnip greens, romaine, baby gems, and Swiss chard. It's also abundant in cruciferous veggies like brussels sprouts, broccoli, cauliflower, and cabbage.

Biotin	Needed during the final trimester of pregnancy to help support the increased metabolic demand both you and your baby are experiencing. It can also help with your energy, mood, and stress levels. Pregnant women need about 30 mcg of biotin daily from whole-food sources.	Egg yolks, nuts and seeds, legumes, salmon, tuna, sweet potatoes, and bananas

Copycat Erewhon White Bean and Kale Salad

Ingredients

    1 large bag shredded kale (slicing kale can be time-consuming,
        so this cuts down on prep time)
    Olive oil and salt
    1 (15-ounce) can cannellini or white beans
    1 avocado
    1 tablespoon maple syrup
    1 tablespoon Dijon mustard
    2 garlic cloves, minced
    Juice of 2 lemons
    Freshly ground pepper
    2 tablespoons apple cider vinegar
    1/3 cup hemp hearts

1. Massage kale with olive oil and a generous amount of salt. This step is key. Massaging the kale with oil and salt makes it super tender and allows it to soak up alllll the dressing.
2. Drain and rinse the cannellini beans.
3. Chop the avocado into cubes.
4. In a separate bowl, mix the maple syrup, Dijon mustard, garlic, juice of two lemons, pepper, apple cider vinegar, and hemp hearts.

5. Combine the kale, beans, avocado, and maple syrup mixture together in one big bowl. If you can stand to wait an hour, let it sit in the fridge. Otherwise, enjoy!

PS: This salad keeps for three days in the fridge and just gets better the longer it sits!

Curried Cauliflower and Sweet Potato Soup

Ingredients

1/4 white onion, chopped

1 tablespoon olive oil

2 cups sweet potato, cubed (Remember! The skin has nutrients, so you don't need to peel them.)

2 cups cauliflower florets

2 garlic cloves, minced

1 stick lemongrass

1-inch knob ginger, grated

2 tablespoons curry powder

2 cups vegetable broth

Salt and pepper to taste

Sour cream or coconut yogurt for garnish

Cilantro for garnish

Toasted sunflower seeds for garnish

1. In a large saucepan, sauté onion in olive oil until translucent (again, one of the best smells in the world).
2. Add in the sweet potato, cauliflower, garlic, lemongrass, ginger, curry powder, and vegetable broth.
3. Raise the heat and bring to a simmer, cooking until cauliflower and sweet potato are tender (about 30 minutes).

4. Remove the lemongrass and use an immersion blender to blend the ingredients to a smooth consistency. A regular blender works just as well; you'll just need to be careful when pouring the soup into the blender.
5. Add salt and pepper if needed.
6. Top with sour cream (or coconut yogurt), cilantro, and toasted sunflower seeds!

SIXTEEN

LET'S HEAR IT FROM THE DAD

I've said a lot of nice things about Daryl in this book, and even though every word of it is true, it's not the full truth: he's actually even better in person. I didn't tell you guys that when we found a breakfast that didn't spike my blood sugar, he cooked it for me every morning and delivered it to me in bed (a.k.a. the couch). I *did* tell you that he rubbed my feet every single night and never missed a chance to tell me I was beautiful. I left some things out because honestly, Daryl raises the bar and some people find it annoying to read about a perfect partner. So why am I putting it in the book now? Because Daryl is amazing, and he raises the bar . . . but it's a bar that everyone else should meet, TBH. Having a loving, supportive partner who is *in this pregnancy with you* is what everyone deserves. You deserve to feel like your partner is truly your partner in this pregnancy, even though it's happening in your body.

So for this chapter, I'm handing it over to Daryl to let him speak for himself (and to any partners out there who want to know how to step it up during pregnancy).

Daryl Says

I grew up without a dad, the son of a single mother. Maybe that's why I never really saw myself being a dad: it's hard to see yourself in a role you never had modeled for you outside of movies. Lucky for me, I was raised by rom-coms, and the dads I loved on-screen—Tom Hanks in *Sleepless in Seattle* and Michael Keaton in *Mr. Mom*—were fun and loving and present with their kids. As a kid, that's exactly the kind of dad I wanted: a dad who talked to me, listened to me, played with me, showed me that they cared about me. As an adult, I just assumed that kids and marriage weren't for me . . . and then I met Meghan. I knew on our first date that she was the one and that whatever she wanted, I wanted. Within a few weeks, we were talking about marriage, and even though I'd never seen myself as a potential dad, with her it made sense. Of course we'd have kids. We were going to be a family.

To be honest, a huge part of that is Meghan's family. I know not everyone is blessed with in-laws that they love, but I am. The Trainors are close (I mean, as she's mentioned, her brothers live with us) and loud and hilarious. They love one another really intensely; they put one another first; they're real and honest with one another. I didn't just want to be a part of that, I wanted to build on it.

Marriage is a partnership, and so is building your family. Anything that Meghan and I do together feels like we're in it together, all the way. I don't think I did anything special during Meghan's pregnancy . . . until I hear from other people that it's unusual for a guy to be this involved. And honestly, it makes me sad. This is a short time in both your lives, a truly incredible part of life, and something you're lucky to be able to share with the person you love. Being a dad is a privilege, and even though Riley has made our lives 1 million percent more fun, it's a privilege that I take really seriously.

The misconceptions about pregnant women are that they're *crazy* and *hormonal* and yeah, Meghan may have had a moment or two, but I stood in awe of her throughout this experience. The mother of your children is allowed to be emotional; she's allowed to struggle. Talk to her about what she's feeling, and why. Or sometimes, don't talk…just listen! Do some research on what's happening inside her and how that could be affecting her. I know she handed you this chapter of the book, but go through and read the whole thing (and I'm not just saying that because my wife wrote it). Just do something, without being asked: take care of her, because she's taking care of your child already. Forty weeks is a relatively short time in the grand scheme of things, and this is not an exact experience either of you will ever have again. You'll never be pregnant for the first time again, and even future pregnancies will be different. When I thought about it like that—a finite experience—there was nothing I wouldn't do to make this easier for Meghan.

I don't blame men for feeling lost in this experience; for generations, pregnancy has been "women's business." Our grandpas were in the waiting room while our grandmas gave birth, and I can pretty much guarantee they never went to any doctor's appointments or helped put together a nursery or said "We're pregnant." But lucky for us, it's the twenty-first century, and we have a hand in changing the culture around birth and pregnancy. So if I can offer any dad-to-be advice, it's this:

WORK ON YOURSELF

The strength of my relationship with Meghan is in part because we've worked on ourselves too. We deal with our anxieties and our issues; we each go to therapy. I spend time every day meditating and getting grounded because the better *I* am, the better *we* are. I went sober for Meghan's entire pregnancy: she couldn't drink either, obviously, and I wanted to be as present as possible for the experience.

YOU'RE IN THIS TOGETHER

She's pregnant, but you're *both* having a baby. Whatever anxieties you have about what's to come, remember that she's putting together a whole person inside her. She's forming a skeleton, a little brain, an entire *child* . . . while she's also doing everything else she's always done. The things happening inside her body (and her mind) are not anything you can relate to, so double the normal amount of love and compassion you have for her. I looked at Meghan every single day like she was a god: she was growing our child, and the least I could do was make her breakfast.

What she cares about, you should care about. It doesn't matter whether it's baby clothes or the birth plan: if she's googling it, you should too. When Meghan asked me to pack her hospital bag, I did my own research and came up with a list. I bought three different kinds of maternity panties so she could have options and tell me what she liked. I saw a TikTok of a guy who brought a PlayStation to the hospital while his wife was in labor because "there was nothing else for him to do." Dude. There's plenty for you to do. Be present. Hold her hand. Go get her ice. Text updates to your family. If you really think that the best use of your time when your wife is having a baby is to be playing a video game with your buddies, I feel bad for your wife and I feel bad for your kids. This is the one time she will be in labor with this baby, so show up fully.

YOU'RE HERE TO LEARN

Whatever kind of dad you had—or didn't—you get to decide the kind of father you want to be. You get to break generational curses and change your family tree, or pass down the best parts of your own dad to your children. Movies about fatherhood usually feature some kind of freak-out by the guy; in *She's Having a Baby*, Kevin Bacon has a meltdown; in *Knocked Up*, Seth Rogen freaks out . . . but I never felt that panic about what was to come, even though I hadn't had a father. You can read all the books and watch all the YouTube videos, but parenthood requires on-the-job training. I'd never held a baby or changed a diaper or mixed a bottle. Instead of letting myself feel dumb or helpless, I took it all as an opportunity for growth. Meghan had always been baby crazy, but we both became parents at the same time. She'd held babies, but never *our* baby. She'd changed diapers, but never *Riley's* diaper. It can be a really cool experience to learn alongside your partner and to learn these new versions of yourself and each other. I met—and fell in love with—Meghan all over again as a mom. For my first Father's Day, she made a video of Riley and me. She'd captured all these tiny moments: making him laugh, rocking him, dancing around the kitchen to his mom's music. It was just a few minutes long, but it showed me that the kind of dad I am is the kind of dad I always dreamed of having.

It's true that as soon as you master one phase of parenting, your kid moves on to another. There will always be more to learn as Riley and our family grow, and I'm sure I'll make plenty of mistakes. In my experience, I'm learning fatherhood from Riley: he is teaching me every day about what he needs, leading me toward this new version of myself. Learn from your partner and your child. Let this experience grow you. And for fuck's sake, don't bring a PlayStation to the hospital.

SEVENTEEN

HERE COMES RILEY

Surrender became my mantra, and with that surrender, I felt less fear and more excitement. Don't get me wrong—I was fucking terrified about that surgery, but I was excited that I knew exactly when we were going to meet our baby. I wouldn't be waking Daryl up in the middle of the night or racing to the hospital. The countdown became epic for the whole family. We made a countdown on the calendar in our bathroom and every day we'd cross off another number and say, "Nine days until we meet the baby!" "Eight days until we have our baby!" "Seven days until I have this baby!"

The last week was torture, not just because I was excited to meet him but because I was in so much pain. I felt like my stomach was going to explode and I couldn't stand without my feet feeling like they were on fire. I complained any time I had to take a few steps. We were all placing bets on how big the baby would be. I thought he'd be at least nine pounds. Daryl had been packing the hospital bag for forever, and every day packages from Amazon arrived. The pandemic was raging and we were afraid to go anywhere, and every day I saw a new YouTube video about "what I *really* used in the hospital." Let me tell you this:

I learned absolutely nothing. They were all wrong. I love influencer content, but it's designed to sell you an aesthetic, and childbirth is not aesthetic, y'all. Maybe I'm just jealous, but I'm not the kind of person who is going to pack multiple outfits for a surprise outfit change. But watching all this stuff made me *want* to be that person, and so I bought a ton of stuff that I absolutely didn't need. The only things in my bag that I'm glad I had were a blanket and a pillow, because I'm picky. Every person and each pregnancy are so different that trying to get advice about what you will want for an experience you've never had before is useless. Besides, the hospital will have what you truly *need*. That's kind of their job.

EVERYTHING YOU DON'T NEED
FOR THE HOSPITAL

I rolled up to the hospital with two suitcases, and it was a total waste of space and time. Here's everything I absolutely did not need to bring.

- A cute little fan. I don't know what I thought this would do for me. The temperature was fine; if anything, hospitals are kind of cold.
- Books. You think you're going to read between contractions? No shot.
- Headphones. Uh, what? What are you going to listen to? A podcast? You're alone in a room with your husband, so I guess pack these if you hate him and don't want to hear his voice?
- Outfits. The hospital literally gives you an outfit. It's a little hospital gown and it's accessible and comfy and nobody cares what you look like. They even give you cozy socks with grips.
- A razor. Who cares if your legs or pits are hairy? *You just had a baby!*

- **A loofah.** The bathroom is not big enough to have a relaxing shower.
- **Pajamas.** I lived in my hospital gown, and honestly, I didn't care what I was wearing.
- **Multiple outfits for your baby.** Your baby needs *one* outfit to go home in.
- **Gifts for your baby.** Your baby doesn't care about presents yet.
- **A cute robe.** Again, I wore just the hospital gown. And robes take up a lot of room!
- **Makeup.** Who cares what you look like? *You just had a baby!* I say this as a person who loves glam, but I could not be bothered to put a drop of makeup on my face after having a baby, and my husband couldn't possibly have cared less. I had nobody to impress and no desire to put makeup on.

When February 8 rolled around, we woke up feeling more excited and nervous than we ever had in our lives. This was like Christmas morning in February. We were going to meet our baby today! My C-section was scheduled for noon, but I had to get there two hours early like I was taking a flight. We hugged my family goodbye, and I told everyone, "Next time I see you I'll have a baby!" I was feeling excited and strong even though I couldn't believe I was going to have a baby without my mom there. My mom is my best friend (sorry, Daryl), and I do everything with her. I always imagined her there by my side when I became a mom, but instead she just walked me to the car and waved goodbye with tears in her eyes while we drove off to officially become parents.

Instead of the frantic drive to the hospital that you see in movies, where the woman is screaming and the man is dripping sweat, we rolled into the hospital with our packed suitcases like we were leaving to go on vacation, ready to meet our baby. If you're imagining this as a glamorous moment . . . nope. When we pulled into the parking lot, we were a mess: the car door nearly shut on my head while I was trying to help Daryl pull out our luggage, and we were so visibly nervous that the couple parking next to us stopped and asked if it was our first time. They were heading in for their *third* C-section, and it didn't look like they were moving in. The mom told us—so nicely—that we didn't need to bring in all our stuff right away, just what I actually wanted with me in the room for the procedure. Thank God they were there, or I'd have walked in with an empty stroller and a car seat. They were so comforting; they walked in so naturally that it made us feel less nervous. They were like undercover angels for our special day.

Walking into the hospital was like stepping up to a counter to order lunch.

"Hi, I'm Meghan, I'd like a C-section today."

"Of course. Have a seat and we'll be right with you."

They walked us down the hall to our room, and a woman rushed by us in full-on labor, screaming and clutching her belly and back. Very chill and not at all stressful. Honestly, it made me glad I wasn't going to go into labor. I'd just get numbed up, lie down, and get my baby.

In our little room, there was a bed but no shower. I was a little freaked out, thinking I would be here for the next few days, but, you know, *surrender*. But that was just the room where I got my IV while they prepared the surgical room and checked to make sure I wasn't having contractions. My nurse heard my entire life story, and I asked her a million questions about her life. It's so funny to think that these people are a part of the most important moments of your life and you never see them again, but I think of them like guardian angels. She made me feel totally comfortable and even took a photo of me and Daryl together, telling us, "This is the last photo of the two of you before you become parents!" It was time for the biggest moment of our lives, and all we had to do was just walk down the hallway to the surgical room. The entire experience is so surreal: it's a huge deal and no big deal all at once.

I went in alone to get my epidural, which is basically a huge needle that goes into your spine to numb you from the ribs down. I'd seen a ton of YouTube videos and Instagram posts where people freak out about this, but it really wasn't that bad. *Surrender*, I told myself. But then they asked whether it was okay for the residents to do my epidural, and for the first time in my life I stood up for myself. I love doctors, and a teaching hospital is an incredible thing, but I was not comfortable with anyone learning on me during my first C-section.

When the (very young) doctor walked in, I didn't think about the giant needle; I just distracted myself by cracking jokes about how young he looked. He was a very good doctor, and I'm sorry if I hurt his feelings, but I was nervous. He looked so young I thought they may have ignored my request, but he assured me he was fully qualified.

I loved being in a room of (mostly) women, and I reminded myself that if anything felt weird, I'd say something. I had a shooting pain down my right leg and immediately told them what was happening, and they adjusted something that made it go away. *Surrender*.

You can't lie on your back while the epidural is kicking in, so I was kind of awkwardly sitting up, asking questions like "Oh my God, what if I pee?" They laughed. I already had a catheter in and didn't even feel it. The epidural was already doing its job. Once I was nice and drugged up, they finally let Daryl come in. He'd been in the hallway listening to a song I wrote for him years before called "You're Worth Waiting For." It's never been officially released, but he had it on his phone and I love him for how sentimental he is.

You're worth waiting for, baby you're worth waiting for
And I'm grateful I ain't got to wait no more
You're worth waiting for

While Daryl was looking at me like I was the most amazing woman on the planet, the doctors started to do their thing. Dr. Solky introduced me to everyone, told me what everyone's job was, and reminded us what we were all here to do: deliver a happy, healthy baby boy. It felt a little bit like being a slab of meat, or an extra in *Grey's Anatomy*. I could hear them confirming all the tools they'd need, even though I couldn't see anything because of the big sheet they put between my head and my torso. I had told the anesthesiologist that I wanted to know when the surgery was beginning. I heard what sounded like a Dremel tool whirling and he looked down at us and said, "Okay, they're starting." Dude. I thought it would be a quiet little slice, not some loud-ass power tools.

I don't want to scare you, so if you're not into the details, skip the next part: you can smell yourself. Like, your burning skin. I'd been warned about that smell, but there is nothing to prepare you for it. It's . . . not a good smell, and it will stick with you for a while. But honestly, I can't remember it now; I just know that it was pungent.

Daryl gripped my hand like I would be pulled away from him. I couldn't feel any pain, but I could feel myself being yanked around down there. Daryl kept me present and grounded.

A C-section is an intense experience: you are fully awake and *know* that someone is opening your body to take out your child, and you can *feel* people pulling and yanking . . . but you can't see a thing. But Daryl could, and he stood by my side for every minute. His eyes locked on mine made me feel safe and alive. On his phone, he played Justin Bieber's "Anyone." This version hadn't come out yet, but we had the demo on my phone from the original writer, and we sang every word to each other, shaking in fear and smiling.

It felt like I was there for hours, but seven minutes and a giant *pop* later, I heard Dr. Solky ask if I wanted to meet my baby. This is a moment that will live in my mind forever. Above the blue curtain that separated my head from the surgical team, a tiny face arrived, perfect and round. He opened one eye, and my heart stopped. It was like when they raised Simba up in *The Lion King*.

"Whoa," I whispered. "He's actually beautiful."

I said *actually* because he didn't look like my cousin had, because he hadn't had to squish through the birth canal. (Bonus for C-section babies: they're extra pretty right away.) He was perfect and gorgeous. Our Riley was here. They whisked him back over the curtain, and after a few minutes I realized that I hadn't heard him cry.

"Why isn't he crying?" I asked, and I saw Daryl's face change as he looked over to where our baby was being worked on by the doctors.

Daryl Says

Everyone who works in a delivery room or the neonatal intensive care unit (NICU) should be an actor. Riley wasn't crying, and you could tell something wasn't right, but everyone was smiling at me and nobody looked worried. Even the guy who was tossing Riley around was smiling while he said, "Usually we'd hear more noise and his breathing is a little shallow." My number one priority was to make sure Meghan got skin-to-skin contact with Riley right away, and it felt like I was failing. She was drugged out of her mind and I didn't want her to worry, so I did my best to try to stay calm.

"It just takes a minute sometimes," they told me, and in my drug haze I just thought, *But I want to hold him.* I really, really wanted to hold him and get skin-to-skin contact right away, but after ten minutes they told us he needed to go to the NICU.

"Can she see him, please?" Daryl asked.

The energy in the room was tense, and someone told me there wasn't time, but that sweet angel of a nurse brought my baby over to me and set his warm little body right on my chest. It was exactly what I'd been dreaming of for all those months. I put my finger on his cheek to make sure this was real and that I was awake. Daryl took a photo, and they whisked him away. I'd held him for maybe six seconds. Daryl's face was panicked, but as freaked out as I felt inside, the drugs I'd been given for the surgery wouldn't let me panic.

"Do you want me to stay with you or go with Riley?" he asked. I had at least forty-five minutes to be "sewed up," so I asked him to stay with me, but the doctor spoke over me.

"Dad," she said, "you should go with your baby." I was devastated. Good thing I was drugged, or I'd have jumped up with a gaping hole in my belly and run right after them.

The drugs kept me from panicking, but they didn't keep my heart from breaking. I was alone, without Daryl or Riley, and I wasn't sure if my baby could even breathe. Would he be okay? Would Daryl be okay, up there on his own with this crisis? The drugs and the stress made it seem like everything was happening in slow motion. I didn't feel pain, but I could feel the sensation of every tool inside me. I felt and heard a suction tool up by my ribs. I could still smell my own burning flesh. I felt nauseous and light-headed, but the moment I mentioned it to the anesthesiologist, he made it go away. Science is crazy.

Daryl had left with both our phones, so there was no more music, just the sound of tools inside my body. My doctor tried to lighten the mood by telling me my insides were beautiful, but I couldn't laugh. I tried to get myself to take a nap to make the time pass faster, but I knew where I was and the reality I was facing, and it was too scary to fall asleep.

When it was over and they put me on a rolling bed to wheel me to my room, I heard the weirdest thing: "All About That Bass" blasting from another surgical room. I was still drugged as hell, so I started dancing with my arms and telling everyone it was my song. My nurse laughed. I guess another mom had heard I was there and blasted my song to help celebrate my delivery. Whoever you are, that was iconic, and I will never forget it. Thank you.

In the recovery room, it was just me and my angel nurse. She was so calm and so reassuring. She called the NICU to check on Riley for me and had them send Daryl down to my room to bring me my phone. He burst into the room and told me, "He's beautiful, he's perfect," and then ran back to the NICU with his phone and FaceTimed me so I could see Riley. He was *not* nine pounds; he was seven pounds, eight ounces. I cried when I saw all the tubes and cords connected to him. He felt so far away. But I was also distracted by his beauty and by the fact that he was a real person out in the world. I couldn't wait to hold him, rock him, nurse him, kiss him.

Surrender, I reminded myself, *surrender.* I was still feeling no pain, and I FaceTimed my family to tell them that having a baby was no big deal . . . except that Riley was in the NICU for respiratory issues. My mom was panicking and tearing up on the phone, but I kept telling her it was "fiiiiiiine!" I think I felt fine because of my nurse. She didn't judge me when I said I was jealous of the couple next door who had their screaming baby in the room with them, or when I got sad because I didn't have photos to send the friends who texted to check in on me, knowing it was the date of our C-section.

This is where I owe that angel nurse a big, huge thank-you. I know I said it about a thousand times while we were in the hospital room, but I can't possibly say it enough. Wherever you are, I hope you know that your presence and your kindness got me through the scariest parts of that day (and frankly, my life). Thank you for getting Riley into my arms, for laughing at my jokes, and for making me feel like everything was going to be okay. Riley was being taken good care of, and so was I.

THE RECOVERY

I imagined spending the days of C-section recovery holding our baby while glowing with joy. But instead, we both spent two days recovering on different floors of the hospital. It was torture to know that he was so close and yet out of my reach. I had blood in my pee (sorry, but it's true) and I had to wait until I was peeing clear to see my son. I chugged that cranberry juice like I was at a frat party, and when my pee was finally clear, Daryl was allowed to wheel me up to the fourth floor. Every single bump ripped through my body like an earthquake, but I had to see my baby.

Daryl wheeled me through a maze of tiny babies with serious medical issues, past families whose babies might not make it home. It was a real reality check. Finally, we saw Riley. He was in an incubator, connected to what looked like hundreds of wires, but I didn't see any of that. I saw our baby—a tiny Daryl—and I was completely in love.

"We have to have more," I told Daryl, slipping my hands into the incubator to feel our son's heartbeat.

This was the first day I got to hold Riley—really hold him—and I didn't want to let go. I took my shirt off and held him against my skin, and felt his little ribs rise and fall under my hand. But those wires snapped me back to reality real quick. It was like a movie. If the heart rate monitor shifted even a little bit, an alarm would blare and I'd feel like he was about to die. The nurses would just push a button and turn it off like it was no big deal, but it's jarring (especially when you're still drugged up).

Every day, Daryl would wheel me up to see our boy, and we'd spend hours looking at him, singing to him, and eventually holding him. He was so small, and there were so many cords, we both felt like we'd break him if we picked him up. But he was surprisingly sturdy for a tiny little guy, and holding him was absolute heaven.

I would have spent every minute in the NICU, but I had my own healing to do. Standing up and sitting down were even harder than they'd been when I was at the end of my pregnancy. Daryl would help lower me to and hoist me off the toilet, and he would take me for little walks, cheering me on and telling me how strong I was. I didn't feel strong. I used to do actual workouts, and now I felt like a champion if I could walk down the hallway? Mentally, I felt like the C-section scar could open up at any minute and all my guts could spill out. And then it happened. Or, it felt like it happened. I plopped onto the toilet to take my first pee after delivery and I felt something fall out of me. Something big. Something that made a splash.

I was freaking the fuck out, telling the nurse "I think something bad is happening." She was freakishly calm and said, "You're fine; it's normal." When I finally got up, there was a big-ass blood clot sitting in the bowl. I knew you could bleed after a vaginal birth, but I was not prepared for this to happen after a C-section. It seriously felt like I'd lost an organ, but apparently it was no big deal? Our bodies are amazing and crazy.

POST C-SECTION REVIEWS

Everyone—and their recovery—is different, but here were the absolute worst parts for me:

- **Pumping:** The first thing I had to do when I got to my room was use a breast pump. I was shocked because I'd heard it takes a few days for your milk to come in, but apparently pumping helps it come in. I had no idea what I was doing. I asked the nurse if it was supposed to hurt so bad and she said, "Yeah, it's supposed to be uncomfortable." Wrong. After twenty minutes my left areola was bleeding and raw. Every three hours, I still had to do this, even though it was absolute misery and I was exhausted. 0/5 stars.
- **The pain:** I'd told everyone that having a baby was no big deal and it didn't hurt . . . until it did hurt. When the pain came in it hit *hard*; I'd never had any kind of surgery or physical trauma, and it felt unbearable. I didn't have a baby to hold and distract me, so I really felt it. 1/5 stars.

- **Peeing:** With a catheter, I loved peeing. I am lazy, and I could just lie there and pee? Heavenly. But once the catheter is out, a nurse has to watch you pee for the first time (seriously). And I couldn't do it. Like, physically the catheter had made my body forget how to pee. It felt like it took fifteen minutes for me to even get a little tinkle, and the pain from the C-section made my body shake uncontrollably. Plus, you know, that blood clot came out while I was peeing. 2/5 stars.
- **Wearing a diaper:** If it weren't for the pain of trying to take it on and off, I probably would have actually liked this. Again, I'm lazy, and the diaper was kinda comfortable. 3/5 stars.

RILEY'S RECOVERY

The NICU is a really special place. No parent ever expects that their child will be there, but the people who work there have dedicated their lives to helping these little babies survive and thrive. It was hard, though. He'd been inside me for thirty-nine weeks and now we were separated by a few floors in a hospital. We weren't sure how long he'd be there, but there were a lot of babies in the NICU who were really struggling, and Daryl and I felt blessed knowing that what Riley was going through was survivable. There's a solidarity among the parents in the NICU. The energy is quiet and low, and we didn't speak to the other parents, but we'd all give one another the look and the nod as we walked by. *I see you.*

We would get to bring our baby home soon, and not all of the parents in the NICU would get to do that. We didn't have a clear timeline on when, though. "It's up to Riley" seemed to be the reply, and that was not a very satisfying answer. I wanted to be told a date and a time when his respiratory issues would clear up and he'd be good to go. *Surrender,* I tried to remind myself, *surrender.*

Our pediatrician came to meet Riley the day after he was born and assured us that a lot of babies go through this and that Riley would make progress and come home to us. It took five days in the NICU to finally get Riley cleared to come home. Five days of visits where he was covered in cords and tubes, and where I had to stay in a wheelchair. As much as possible, we held him to our chests, skin to skin, and talked to him. On his last night, we begged for him to be able to stay with us in our room so we could have a practice run at life as a family of three. We learned to change him, bathe him, swaddle him. We all snuggled in the hospital bed together and talked about how beautiful he was. And the next morning, we packed our bags and headed home.

TRIMESTER FOUR

EIGHTEEN

IT'S NOT OVER . . . IT'S JUST BEGINNING

The first time I heard about the "fourth trimester," I thought someone just counted wrong. The fourth trimester of pregnancy is your first three months of motherhood, a time of huge growth for your baby *and* for you. You've been plunged into a new role and identity, you're learning as you go, and you're still healing. We live in a culture that is obsessed with hustle and productivity, and I get it . . . if you're a doer, it's hard to be *doing* things that aren't measurable. A few weeks ago, you might have been the star of your team at work, and now you're excited that your baby slept for a four-hour stretch. The transition to motherhood can be hard and weird and kind of lonely, especially if you don't have a lot of mom friends around. I was the first mom in my group, and everyone really tried to get excited about Riley's sleep schedule, but it's one of those "if you know, you know" kind of situations.

The next few months are going to go so slow and so fast all at once. On good days, you'll think there isn't a better mom than you, that life is amazing, that you've never been happier. On bad days, you'll be overwhelmed and wondering who the hell let you leave the hospital with a baby when you don't know what you're doing. From every mom I know, that's totally normal. My mom still thinks it's hilarious that *she* is a mother and was responsible for three lives! Your body and your mind have just been through something incredible and intense and maybe traumatic, and as much as we all want to prove that we can do it all, I hope that you take the time to *take your time* this trimester. I know, I know, this is coming from the most impatient woman on the planet, so learn from some of my mistakes, okay?

BRINGING HOME RILEY

It took us a long hour to finally be discharged from the hospital, and it felt like we were springing Riley from baby prison. Before we left, we had to make a bottle with the formula we were encouraged to order from Germany that was the highest, "best" quality of formula you could get. Expensive as fuck, but Riley eventually loved it. One problem: the instructions were *all in German*. We looked at the nurses and asked them to teach us how to make a bottle for our baby and the weirdest thing happened. They said, "Oh, we can't legally help you with outside formula." We were flabbergasted. Luckily, Daryl is a YouTube king like me and figured it out, but it was bizarre and annoying. We brought up the car seat and asked the nurses to help us strap him in perfectly. We filled out a mountain of paperwork, and we waited for a wheelchair so we could finally—finally!—get home. I sat in the back seat next to Riley's car seat, and we took the longest car ride of my entire life. Traffic was still light because of COVID, but it felt like every bump in the road was personally attacking my son and my wound, and I could feel my heart pumping until we safely pulled into our driveway.

Finally, we were home, as a family of three . . . with my entire family waiting inside for us. (In case you're wondering, no, we were not done with the house, and as I'm writing this, we're still not done. Nobody told me the water was off today until *after* I used both toilets. Not cool!) My mom had put up signs that said "Welcome home, baby boy!" and bought Riley a giant stuffed giraffe that I'd wanted ever since I knew I wanted kids (so, forever). One by one, I watched each family member hold our son. All of us were deliriously happy; he was like a little trophy that we couldn't stop passing around. I kept saying "Look at him!" Like anyone could take their eyes off him. Riley was now the center of our universe, and seeing the people I love fall in love with him was a feeling I'll never forget.

Everything felt special that first day at home. I was excited when Riley peed right through his little outfit because I got to take him to our changing table for the first time. We'd set up a little nursery area in our bedroom, and it was finally time to actually use all the stuff we got, to do the simple little things that we'd been dreaming about for months. The high of leaving the hospital had made even a diaper change feel like a big event. I laid him on the changing pad I'd picked out for him, I wiped his little butt with the wipes we'd had delivered, and I couldn't believe that I was changing my own baby's diaper in my own house, with my own mom right next to me. I'd missed her so much while we were in the hospital, and it was so special to have her by my side again . . . especially when Riley had a blowout. I was so delirious and happy about everything, even his dirty diapers. My mom and I examined his ugly, nasty belly button scab like it was the most beautiful thing we'd ever seen.

I spent that whole first day at home running around the house, doing dishes like I hadn't just had surgery. I was high on life, and my extra-strength Tylenol was doing its job, so I was walking around doing the most. I was warned by someone that this might happen with my excitement and adrenaline and that I would regret it at night when the pain finally crept back in—and they were right.

When we lie down to go to sleep that night, it felt like my body was ripping apart. I hadn't been able to feel the surgery when it was happening, but the healing I could feel, and it freaked me out. There was a bandage on my belly that I couldn't even stand to look at, a small wound that they somehow had gotten an entire baby out of. I couldn't think about it without feeling sick, but every time I moved my body, I was reminded of what happened. You know that patience is not my strong suit, but I had a lot of healing left to do.

The recovery for my C-section was supposed to take weeks, plural. Writing this, I think, *Yeah, of course, they sawed you open, babe.* But at the time I thought, *I want to do things around the house; I want to go for long walks as a family; I want to work out!* The first month at home with Riley, our schedule was just a never-ending loop of the same activities:

- Give Riley a bottle.
- Change Riley.
- Sleep.
- Go to the pediatrician. (We went three times in the first week, which was miserable for a girl who just had intense surgery.)
- Try to breastfeed.
- Pump.
- Take Tylenol and cry about the pain.

One thing you'll hear a lot is "Sleep when the baby sleeps!" We never did. We *should* have. But we didn't. We were too excited to be home with my family. I regret not taking those opportunities. Have you ever pulled an all-nighter? That delirious hangover is how you are gonna feel for three months. And they expect us to take care of an infant while feeling like that. It's aggressive, and I wish we had slept while the baby slept. Next baby, I'm going to be sleeping as much as I can, whenever I can.

The physical recovery was really painful. I wanted to be fine and do everything myself, but everything from my ribs to my vag hurt in the weeks after we brought Riley home. If I forgot to take my Tylenol, the pain would get so bad that my teeth would chatter. But I was totally unprepared for how the C-section would affect me mentally. As soon as the sun went down, the pain would creep back up on me and torture me until I fell asleep. Some nights I would cry myself to sleep in pain while Daryl tried to comfort me.

C-SECTION ADVICE I SHOULD HAVE TAKEN

Take it easy. For real, you just had a major surgery. I was running around playing hostess when I should have been healing. Slow down, mama. This goes for any kind of birth, by the way. Sit down. Lie down. Let people wait on you like the queen you are.

Use your pillow! Pressing a pillow against your incision site when you're getting up, sitting down, or about to laugh, cough, or even sneeze will give you extra support and help you not feel like your body is going to rip apart.

Stay ahead of the pain. Again, this goes for any kind of birth. I would forget to take my Tylenol and then be side-swiped by pain. Stay ahead of the pain by staying on top of your meds. Set a timer in your phone if you need a reminder!

After two weeks, I noticed the tape covering my C-section scar was creasing in, and it made my entire body cringe. This was the hole where they took our son out of my body, and the only thing covering it was this tape. I sent photos to Dr. Solky in a panic, and she told me we could take the tape off. Was she crazy? I was terrified. Daryl was ready to be my doctor and rip that bitch off, but I needed a couple more days. Finally, I let him do it. I stood in front of my couch because I was dizzy with panic, thinking I might faint. My knees collapsed as he was ripping it off, and I started freaking out and crying, saying, "slower" and "ahhhhh!" Daryl peeled off the tape gently and slowly while I cried and shook. I was sure the incision would pop open and everything would come falling out. Remember, I'd never had stitches and my medical experience is that I've watched every season of *Grey's Anatomy*.

"Is it bleeding? Is it bleeding?" I was sweating and frozen in fear with my pants down like a toddler having a meltdown.

"No," he said with a laugh. "It's incredible."

I thought he was crazy for saying it was incredible, but he really was the best doctor and hubby for me in that moment. He knew exactly what to say to calm me down and convinced me that it was the most beautiful scar ever and that I was healing so well.

CONTENT WARNING: SKIP THIS NEXT PARAGRAPH IF YOU DON'T WANT TO BE FREAKED OUT ABOUT A C-SECTION. THIS WAS JUST *MY* EXPERIENCE, AND YOURS COULD BE TOTALLY DIFFERENT!

Nighttime was the worst, and not just physically. When it was quiet and dark, just as I was falling asleep, I'd flash back to the surgery. It was like sleep paralysis: I could sense and feel the surgery all over again, like I was back on the table unable to move. I'd moan and cry and wake up to Daryl asking me what was wrong, and it felt crazy to say, "I was reliving the surgery; it felt real." I would cry and say, "I feel hands inside me."

Because of my mental health history, I'd been vigilant about watching for postpartum depression and postpartum anxiety. I somehow didn't get either one, but what I was experiencing was post-traumatic stress disorder. When my therapist said it, I thought, *No, no, I didn't go to* war. *I had a baby.* But, she explained, it wasn't just "having a baby" but the trauma of having Riley ripped away from me and sent up to the NICU with Daryl while I lay helpless on a table hearing—and smelling—my body being put back together. I had called my family and told them it was "no big deal," but my brain was telling me that it was, actually, a very big deal.

I'm so grateful that my therapist identified what was happening to me and that I had access to the care I needed to work through it. Without her, I probably would have just told myself to suck it up and get over it, that I got the baby I dreamed of and I should stop being so negative.

Girl, you cannot think yourself out of a mental health issue. If you feel off, tell someone. Tell your partner. Tell your provider. In the check-ups after you give birth, your provider will screen you for postpartum depression and postpartum anxiety. I'm so grateful they do that. They'll ask you all kinds of questions, and I really hope you'll tell the truth. Getting help is never a sign of weakness, and it is never a sign that you are a bad mom. Postpartum depression affects around one in seven women,[1] and many women don't speak up because they don't want their families to know. Maybe they're afraid of judgment; maybe they're afraid they'll lose support. This is why I tell everyone my business: because the more we talk about it, the more normalized it becomes. The best moms I know are not flawless moms who have never struggled. Those moms don't exist. Even people whose lives look picture-perfect on Instagram are still people, and nobody gets through life without suffering. Life is hard whether or not you're a mom, but when you're responsible for a whole-ass person that you love more than anything in this world? It's a lot. Please please please please *please* take care of yourself and ask for help.

BRINGING YOUR BABY HOME

Life as a family of three is different, and just like pregnancy and birth, you don't really know what you need until you get in there and live it.

Before you bring your baby home, talk with your partner about how you see the first weeks at home going. A few things to think about:

Your guest policy. Honestly, if you can hold out on having guests over for the first month, I would. People are, of course, really excited to meet the new baby. But we learned really quickly that as much as we loved sharing Riley with the people we loved, having guests knocked us on our asses. Part of this was because I kept insisting that I could do everything myself. And I would do everything except the two most important things: feeding myself and taking my medicine. Of course, I'd start shaking in pain and feel light-headed AF. Come up with some boundaries around visitors and communicate them clearly: "Saturday works for us. Could you come by from nine to nine thirty?" Giving people a clear window of time will keep you from becoming a hostess when you really should be sitting back like a queen and be waited on. If people don't get the hint that it's time to go, here's a trick: stand up and say, "It was so great of you to stop by; I'm going to go lie down, but let's do this again soon." If they don't get *that* hint, well, your partner is going to have to handle it because you'll already be in your room with the baby.

Let people help. You cannot—I repeat, cannot—do everything on your own. So for these next three months (and as long as you have people asking what they can do), let people help you. Your mom wants to unload the dishwasher? Great. Let her do it! The neighbor wants to mow the lawn? Fantastic, have them fire up the mower and come on over. Your best friend wants to bring you dinner and hold the baby so you can take an hour-long shower? Amazing, tell her exactly what you're craving. Just because you *can* do something doesn't mean you have to do it on your own, and the people who love you really do want to know how to help. If someone comes over to visit and you need help folding baby laundry, ask them to do it with you. If you need them to hold the baby so you can use the bathroom, say it. And if someone says, "Let me know what I can do," trust that they mean it. I know this is a scary idea; my generation is afraid to make a phone call, let alone make a request of somebody. But try it! Be specific about what you need and when you need it:

- Hey, you mentioned having some time to help out. Could you walk our dog tomorrow morning before ten?
- I need someone to wait for the fridge repair guy while I take the baby to the pediatrician; could you be at our house from ten to twelve on Saturday?

Most people will jump at the chance to be told exactly how to help, and if they can't help with *that* task, maybe they'll volunteer to do something else.

It's not in reach for most people, but if you *can* hire help, do it. Having a nanny or a night nurse or a house cleaner doesn't make you less capable or less of a mother. With all the family members I have, we didn't need extra help. Also, COVID terrified me and I didn't want to test someone every day and have them in and out of my house. We actually waited until Riley was fifteen months old to get extra help. We were terrified and lost. But now that we've found the *one*, we can't imagine life without her and don't know how we survived a day without her. It was truly a game changer.

Teamwork. At this point, you know that Daryl was—and is—a great partner, but we still had to learn how to do everything together. He jumped right in and did everything for me or alongside me. If I was pumping or trying to nurse, he was right there next to me with the nipple shields ready to go. He didn't just change Riley's diapers, he changed *my* diapers. He didn't just bathe Riley, he helped bathe me in the shower. In the first few weeks, when Riley was eating every two hours, he got up with me. This is just how our marriage is, but I know it's not the case for a lot of couples. *Talk about it.* Talk about it now, before the baby gets here. There's a lot you won't know until the baby arrives, but here's what everyone knows: it's a lot of work. If your partner has never changed a diaper or fed a baby, how do they feel about it? What kind of a parent do they imagine themselves being?

Daryl Says

Dads and partners: Now that the baby is here, it's your time to shine. If you felt like there wasn't really anything you could do while she was pregnant, now there is *plenty* to do. If you see something that needs doing, do it. You might do it wrong, but at least it got done, and you can learn when she tells you that actually, the diaper you put on is on backward. These first few months especially can be painful and overwhelming for her, so if you're not sure what to do, do this:

- Bring her food and water while she's feeding the baby. Any finger foods that are easy to grab with one hand are ideal.
- Remind her to eat—she will forget—and make her favorite foods.
- If she had a C-section or needed stiches, remind her to take her pain medicine; she *will* forget.
- Download any and all apps that help you track this stuff. We live in the future.
- Put the baby monitor on your side of the bed and get up when the baby cries.
- Be the gadget dad and hook up every device to your phone and your wife's phone.
- Pay attention to the baby products that work best for your family and stock up.
- Tell her she's doing an amazing job and that she's hot AF.
- Ask her what you can do better . . . and listen to the answer.
- Say sorry, even if you're certain you weren't wrong. (You probably were wrong.)

NINETEEN

FOURTH-TRIMESTER FOOD AND FITNESS

Keep It Moving with Rebecca ————

You might be in a rush to "get your body back," but you never lost it: your body just went through an incredible journey, and this period of your life is about celebration, not punishment. Our culture puts so much pressure on moms to "snap back," and if you need to go on a social media fast to protect your mental health from seeing messages like that, do it! Because *you just made a whole person, and we don't need to judge our beautiful bodies for looking like they did just that.*

If you're itching to get back to putting in the work, I get it, but we have to make sure it is done properly and safely! The first three months of your baby's life is intense; you're adjusting to huge changes in your body and your schedule, and it can be overwhelming. Be as gentle with yourself in this period as you were in the first trimester. There's no rush to go and run a marathon or try to set a deadlift record. Ease into working out and give your body time to rest and recover. You—and your babe!—need it.

A *lot has changed* in your body, so make sure to talk to your doctor about things like diastasis recti—separation of the abs, as we talked about before—and your pelvic floor health. You might need specific interventions to help you heal, so check with your doctor and get cleared for exercise before you attempt anything new. Aim for 8 to 10 reps, unless your body tells you to stop.

Equipment Needed:

Dumbbells (5-to-8-pound weights or whatever you feel
   comfortable with)

Glute band

Resistance band

Chair

Fitness mat

Your Affirmation:

I'm amazing, and I'm healing.

Fourth-Trimester Fitness

IF YOU'RE RECOVERING FROM DIASTASIS RECTI

- Skip exercises like sit-ups and crunches or anything that will put pressure on your belly and push your abdominals outward.
- Avoid lifting anything heavier than your new little one.
- When getting out of bed or sitting up, roll onto your side first and use your arms to help push yourself up instead of sitting straight up, which puts way too much strain on your abdomen.

SET 1

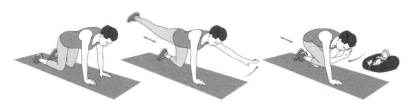

Bird Dog

Start in a tabletop position on your hands and knees. Lift one leg off of the ground straight behind you, simultaneously lifting the opposite arm and reaching as far forward as you can. Exhale as you bring that elbow and knee toward each other, then extend that arm and leg back out and repeat for additional reps. Move to the other side when finished.

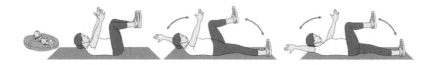

Alternating Dead Bug

Lie on your back with your knees up in a 90-degree angle and your arms straight up in the air. Lower one arm down above your head while keeping it straight, simultaneously extending the opposite leg straight out. Bring the arm and leg back to the starting position, then do the same thing with the opposite arm and leg. Repeat and alternate sides as you go.

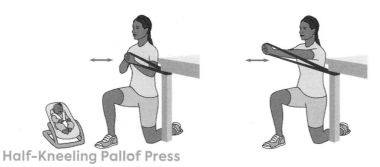

Half-Kneeling Pallof Press

Attach the resistance band to something sturdy, like a heavy table. Start by half kneeling, one knee up and one knee down next to the resistance band. Make sure the leg farther away from the resistance band is the leg that is up and that the band has some resistance when you pick it up and hold it with both hands in front of your chest. "Press" your arms out by straightening/extending them to the front, and then bring them straight back in. Exhale on each press, engaging your core and pelvic floor. Inhale on each pull, lengthening your pelvic floor and breathing into your rib cage. Repeat for additional reps, then switch to the other side.

SET 2

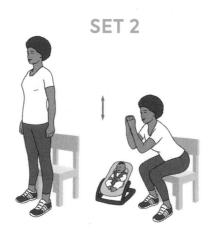

Chair Squat

Standing in front of the chair, engage your core and your pelvic floor. Slowly sit down in the chair and stand back up again to "reset" before repeating.

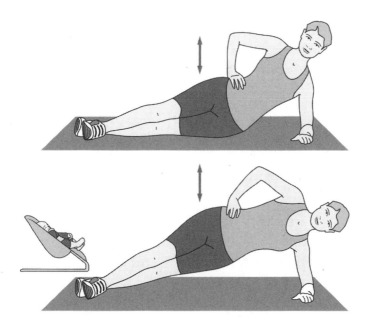

Modified Side Plank

Start by sitting on one side, with one butt cheek on the ground and the arm on that side placed on the floor right next to you. Keeping your knees stacked with your bottom knee on the ground, lift your hips off the ground, making sure your body is in a straight line from the top of your head down to your knees. While engaging your core and your pelvic floor muscles, hold this position for 20 to 30 seconds, then switch and do the opposite side.

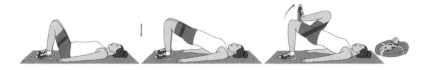

Glute Bridge March

Placing the glute band around your thighs, lie on your back with your hands down by your sides and your feet flat on the ground. Lift your hips up in the air, engaging your pelvic floor muscles and your core. While holding this position, lift one knee up toward your chest and lower it back down. Repeat with the opposite side. Alternate sides for additional reps.

Let's Eat with Kristy

Food is so much more than just food. It's how we nourish and heal ourselves. And now that you're a new mom, it's as important as ever to make sure you're nourishing your body with nutrient-dense foods. If you're nursing, what you eat is also what helps feed your baby's growth and development. But you're *busy*, and in this trimester, we're focusing on what's quick, easy, and nutritious.

QUICK AND EASY

Meal-prepping is the best way to put your nutrition on autopilot and save your brain from having to think about what's for dinner. (Or breakfast. Or lunch.) If you don't have one already, a veggie chopper makes it easy to cut up tons of veggies. Also a sure way to guarantee you're getting protein, veggies, and healthy fats is a good old sheet-pan meal: throw veggies and a protein on a sheet pan, drizzle with olive oil and your favorite seasonings, and bake until done. It doesn't need to be fancy to get the job done.

Traditional Meal Prep

Many of my clients take a Sunday afternoon and prep one breakfast, lunch, and dinner to last the week for their family. It's the easiest, quickest way to make sure every meal is covered, and if you don't mind eating the same thing for seven days, this is a great option.

Mix-and-Match Meal Prep

If the thought of the same meals for a week is a no-go, consider prepping:

- 2 to 3 proteins
- 2 high-fiber carbohydrates
- 3 to 5 vegetables
- 2 sauces
- Fresh berries and greens

Mix-and-Match Menu	
Proteins	• roasted salmon • crispy chickpeas
Carbohydrates	• brown rice • roasted sweet potatoes
Veggies	• grilled zucchini • grilled bell peppers • steamed broccoli • grilled asparagus • roasted brussels sprouts • roasted mushrooms • whatever veggies you'll actually eat
Sauces	• lemon tahini dressing • store-bought pesto • store-bought red sauce • whatever sauce you love
On hand	• arugula • avocado • berries • yogurt • nut butter

Meal Kits

There are lots of options now for services that will deliver prepped ingredients or ready-to-heat-and-eat meals right to your door. This is a great option for any family, especially when there's a new baby. Many of them offer options for special diets (gluten free, dairy free, etc.).

NUTRIENT-DENSE FOODS

Postpartum nutrition looks a lot like a regular healthy eating plan for my clients. I want you filling up on the following foods to make sure your body is getting the vitamins and minerals it needs to support your recovery.

- Vegetables: leafy greens, carrots, kale, broccoli, cauliflower, brussels sprouts, peppers, tomatoes, celery, cabbage, asparagus, and zucchini
- Fruit: berries, citrus, mango, pineapple, papaya, apples, and bananas
- Complex carbs: oats, sweet potatoes, quinoa, brown rice, and whole-grain bread
- Proteins: salmon, shrimp, chicken, eggs, turkey, grass-fed beef, beans, lentils, and edamame
- Healthy fats: avocado, olive oil, nuts, and seeds
- Dairy (organic whenever possible): yogurt, cottage cheese, and kefir

There are also a few specific nutrients that you should focus on consuming during this time.

What It Is	Why You Need It	Where to Get It
Iodine	It's important for lactating mothers, and you need almost twice as much as you did pre-pregnancy.	Tuna, oysters, shrimp, seaweed, milk, yogurt, cheese, and beef liver. Note that cruciferous veggies (like broccoli, cauliflower, cabbage, and kale) can inhibit iodine absorption, so don't eat them together.
Choline	Plays a critical role in the development of your baby's brain and nervous system. You need more while breastfeeding to help meet your baby's needs.	Egg yolks, fish, animal proteins, cruciferous veggies, nuts, and seeds
Omega-3 fatty acids	Essential for you and your baby and can help reduce the risk of postpartum depression.	Chia seeds, salmon, mackerel, and walnuts

One of my "rules" is that we try to sit down and savor our meals. Well, that easily goes out the window when you've got a newborn baby and your dinnertime is spent changing a diaper or trying to get *them* to eat. Of course I want you to have enjoyment from eating, but I also know that *this is hard* and we're often lucky if we get to take a few bites of something while it's still hot. It won't always be like this, I promise. Your routine will settle, you'll find a rhythm, and in the meantime, you just do the best you can with the time, money, and mental capacity you have at any given moment.

As mothers, it's very easy for us to forget that loving and caring for ourselves is just as important as loving and caring for our families. This is the most important part of my work: to remind all of you that food is not just food but a form of love. We do not need to be perfect, eat perfectly, or cook picture-perfect meals. Especially in these raw few weeks as a new mom, I hope you are easy on yourself and treat yourself with love and kindness.

Kale and Cannellini Bean Soup

Ingredients

    2 tablespoons extra-virgin olive oil
    1 white onion, chopped
    1 large carrot, chopped
    1 head garlic, separated into cloves and minced
    ½ teaspoon red-pepper flakes
    1 tablespoon dried thyme
    1 pound kale, stemmed and torn into bite-size pieces (a bag is fine!)
    Kosher salt and black pepper
    2 (15-ounce) cans of cannellini beans (a.k.a. Great Northern or
        white beans), drained and rinsed. You can also use chickpeas
        (a.k.a. garbanzo beans) if you'd like.

8 cups chicken bone broth (vegetable broth is also fine)

½ cup grated Parmesan cheese, plus more for serving

1 lemon, juiced

1. In a large pot, heat olive oil over medium-low, then add in the chopped onion and carrot.
2. Sauté until slightly softened (about 5 minutes).
3. Add the minced garlic cloves, red-pepper flakes, and thyme. Cook for about 2 or 3 minutes (until it starts to smell really good).
4. Increase the heat to medium, adding the greens and a pinch each of salt and pepper. Cook until the greens are wilted (about 1 to 2 minutes).
5. Add the beans, broth, and ½ cup Parmesan cheese, and bring to a boil.
6. Reduce the heat to a simmer, cover, and cook until the greens are silky and the beans and broth are warmed through (about 10 minutes).
7. Remove from heat and taste. Stir in lemon juice and taste (you won't use all the lemon), and season with additional salt and pepper.
8. Serve with black pepper and grated Parmesan on top.

Salsa Verde Beef and Cauliflower Rice Bowls

Ingredients

2 pounds skirt or flank steak

Kosher salt

Black pepper

3 tablespoons avocado oil, divided

1 cup salsa verde, plus more for serving

2 cups riced cauliflower (pre-made)

1 avocado, sliced, for serving

¼ white onion, diced small, for serving

Chopped cilantro, for serving, optional

Lime wedges, for serving, optional

1. Cut the steak into 4 large, equal pieces and season generously with kosher salt and pepper.
2. Heat a large skillet over medium-high heat with 2 tablespoons avocado oil. When hot, add your steak. You want to sear the beef on both sides until a deep brown crust forms (3 to 4 minutes per side).
3. Transfer the browned beef to a slow cooker and pour 1 cup of salsa verde over the meat.
4. Cook on high for 4 hours, or on low for 6 to 8 hours.
5. Shred the beef with a fork.
6. Prepare the cauliflower rice. Anything pre-made that you just have to heat up is the easiest option, and right now, we want *easy*. If you're up for it or prefer it, you can use regular rice.
7. To serve, combine the cauliflower rice, shredded beef, sliced avocado, and diced onion. I like it with cilantro and a squeeze of lime.

TWENTY

WHAT YOU REALLY NEED

One thing I noticed right away when we brought Riley home: we had waaaaay too much stuff. All those Instagram ads and those scrolls through Amazon and Target had really gotten me. I had piles of cute little outfits that he never wore because he was in a onesie for the first year of his life. I had tons of little stuffed animals that he never played with. I was Ariel from *The Little Mermaid*, with tons of gizmos and gadgets and doodads that I didn't need. I gave bags of it away, donated some of it, and kept what we really loved and used for my future babies.

By the time you get this book, there will probably be thousands of new products I haven't even heard of, and there are lots of influencers out there giving daily updates on the things you *need* to buy. I included some brand names here because I know some people like to know the exact thing I used, but these are my personal recommendations and *not* sponsored content.

FOR BABY

Rocking Bassinet

We went with a Snoo personally, and it was expensive AF, but Riley is a champion sleeper, and I credit the Snoo. It's incredible, and every mama I know also loved it. You can find them used online, and if you're a mom who can afford one new, make sure you pass it on to another mom when you're done. You can even rent them! It basically gently rocks your baby for you and helps them stay asleep. It even senses when the baby is starting to cry and rocks back and forth like a human to help your baby feel loved, all controlled by an app on your phone.

White-Noise Machine

There are tons of these, but we bought the Hatch brand and loved it so much we bought one for our room too. It's a combination of a night-light and a noise machine, and you can control it with an app (so you don't have to sneak into the room and risk waking up the baby to turn it up or down). Every morning Riley loves to touch the top of it to change the color and change the sounds. He's almost two years old and still does it every day. We also believe it helped his circadian rhythm, because every morning we would turn on the bird sounds and at night it would be the white noise. He slept like a champ for us, and by three months, he was sleeping through the night.

Formula Dispenser Machine

There are a few different things like this on the market, and they're not cheap, but when you're exhausted and you can push a button and get a perfectly mixed, warm bottle of formula? It's priceless. I'll get into more detail on my breastfeeding saga later on, but this machine saved our asses *many* times. We tried a bottle warmer, but it took forever. I'd be holding a screaming kid and when the bottle was done it would be too hot or not warm enough.

A Smart Baby Monitor

Obviously we have camera and audio monitors, but a smart monitor let us see his heartbeat and oxygen levels every night. Checking the app was my addiction and helped me feel at ease, knowing if anything happened, there would be a loud alarm going off. It was great, and I can't imagine how parents didn't have this back in the day. I'm the mom who puts my finger near my baby's nose all day long to make sure he's breathing, so you can imagine how nuts I get when he's asleep.

FOR MAMA

Wearable Breast Pump

I loved these, even if I didn't love breastfeeding. The future is here, and it's tucking these into your bra to milk yourself. I used the Elvie brand. Also, I highly recommend this boobie vibrator I found on Amazon for massaging milk ducts. Felt great. Might make your search history weird?

A Variety of Baby Bottles

There are a *lot* of options, and you don't know what your baby will actually like until they arrive. Instead of buying a full set of one brand, I bought one or two bottles from a range of brands. When Riley picked his favorite bottle, then I went all in. We went through three different bottles until he found his perfect match, which was the MAM Easy Start Anti-Colic Baby Bottle (on Amazon).

•

What products work for you and your baby is so personal, but what every baby and mama needs is *help*. Friends, family, *community*. However you build your village, you're going to need to lean on them.

This isn't a sign that you're weak; it's a sign that you know and respect your human limits. The people who throw you a baby shower (if you let them, LOL) are also the people who want to be a part of your life and your baby's. Let them in. You (and your baby) need them.

TWENTY-ONE

FED IS BEST

My mantra for birth was *surrender*, but my mantra for the first few months of Riley's life was *I'm doing my best*. If you're a planner who likes control, these couple of months are going to fuck with you big-time. I'd heard since the beginning of pregnancy that breastfeeding was challenging but the way to go, and I was so excited to do it. It's another example of how amazing our bodies are: a mom's body creates the perfect food for her baby, and as her baby eats, the mother's uterus contracts while she bonds with her baby. Breastfeeding reduces the risk of ovarian and breast cancers in the mother and the risk of diabetes, asthma, and obesity in babies.[1] I was all in: my body would make amazing milk, my baby would love it, and we'd both get all the bonding and health benefits. I also heard you shed weight while breast-feeding, so I was extra excited about that. Everyone in my family was great at breastfeeding, so I thought it would be a genetic thing, like gestational diabetes was.

Well, it's not. At all. The first time I pumped in the hospital was unpleasant, to say the least. My nipples were raw and bleeding; I asked the nurse if it was supposed to hurt this bad, and she said, "Yeah, it's supposed to be uncomfortable; just do it for twenty-five minutes at least." So I kept going because it was for the baby, and that's what a good mom does, right? I'd been adamant about skin-to-skin contact because I knew how important it was for bonding, and the days he spent in the NICU limited the amount we could have. I kept waiting for my milk to come in, dry pumping every three hours for twenty-five minutes. It *sucked*. It wasn't just uncomfortable; it was painful, and it was hard for me not to feel cheated, like if I'd been able to give birth to Riley and plop him right on my chest, maybe milk would have come in way sooner.

It took a week for my milk to come in, and when it did, I was so excited and amazed at my body. The first time those little drops of milk appeared, it felt like I had struck gold. By this point, I didn't believe any milk was inside me, so when it finally showed up, I took pictures of it and sent it to everyone. In the NICU, Riley wouldn't latch, but the hospital had a new method that would attach a little feeding tube from my nipple that would drop breast milk into Riley's mouth as I pumped a little syringe. It was supposed to trick us both into thinking we were breastfeeding successfully, but it was awkward AF and majorly annoying for all of us. I'd hold Riley, and Daryl would aim the tube into Riley's mouth. I mean, we tried, but most of the milk ended up on me, and Riley and I would both end up crying.

Just after we got home, I met with a lactation specialist. It felt like going back to school; I was so excited to learn and get an A-plus and make some milk for Riley. Because of the challenges I was having, she put me on a triple-feed schedule: I'd try to feed him on my boob, then Daryl would give him a bottle of formula while I tried to pump. My boobs hated this. I hated this. Riley hated it. Daryl was fine, but he hated seeing me and Riley so miserable. When I tell you my boobs hated it, I mean they developed blisters. *Blisters!* I was freaking the fuck out, as you can imagine. My lactation specialist told me to sterilize a needle and pop them. I was almost excited, like I got to pop a giant pimple (I love this because I'm fucking disgusting), but this one was more scary without the same joy. Luckily, I didn't feel the popping of these pimples at all and they emptied out and went away and never came back. Apparently, it was thrush, and the only positive of Riley not latching was that it didn't get in his mouth and irritate him. It looked like yellow, crusty boogers on my nipples. (Hi, Grandma. Sorry.) My nipples were building calluses, I guess? Gnarly. It took about a month and a half for them to get stronger, and eventually pumping wasn't as painful.

IF YOU'RE BREASTFEEDING

- Stay hydrated! I carried a gallon jug around with me (and still do).
- You need about three hundred to four hundred more calories. I kept snacks near me at all times.
- What you eat, your baby eats. Alcohol will show up in your breast milk, and you probably don't want your baby catching a buzz. They sell little test strips so you can check the alcohol content of your milk, or you can pump and dump if you have a glass of wine with dinner. Caffeine can also show up in your breast milk, so you might need to cool it on the coffee.
- This is wild, but certain foods can also affect the taste of your breast milk!
- You can tell early on if your baby has any intolerances (common ones are dairy, eggs, peanuts, soy, and gluten).[2] I had a friend who had to go dairy free while breastfeeding so her baby wouldn't have a bad reaction. Babies can't tell us what's wrong, so if you think something is off

with your baby (they're spitting up a lot when they eat, they're really gassy, or they have a rash or hives), call your pediatrician's nurse line right away.

IF YOU'RE BOTTLE-FEEDING

- Make a schedule with your partner. Parenting is teamwork, and one benefit of formula is that baby doesn't need their mama to make it.
- Nursing pillows aren't just for nursing. They're all about ergonomics, and you might be surprised at how your neck and shoulders get jacked up from hunching over a baby, making sure they're actually eating.
- No microwaves! I know they're fast and convenient, but apparently they don't always heat evenly, and that can burn your baby's mouth. We don't want that.
- Keeping the bottles (and all their parts) clean is really important. Make sure every bottle (and your hands) are clean before every feeding. This can be lots of work, especially in those early days, so if anyone stops over and asks what they can do, put them on bottle-washing duty!

I'd imagined buying an extra refrigerator because my boobs would just be gushing out as much milk as my baby wanted, like he was tapping a keg. Instead, we were both being tortured. My boobs were huge and hard because my ducts were clogging. When they weren't clogged, I wasn't making the amount of milk I thought I'd be making. And even with a nipple shield, my nipples were being straight-up abused by Riley. The poor guy couldn't get milk out, and he was *pissed*. He'd thrash his arms, scratch me, bite at me, pull my nipple with his little, strong gums. When he did get a latch, the release of oxytocin was so intense I felt high. But he could rarely ever get a latch. We went to the lactation specialist with a hungry baby and full boobs and, after getting Riley's weight, spent an hour trying to get him to latch. "You poor thing, you're exhausted," she said to me. I could barely keep my eyes open. After an hour of trying, she weighed him again and saw he gained only 0.6 of an ounce. *WTF is that? Nothing.* It was depressing. The constant pumping and bottle-feeding and breastfeeding attempts were taking a toll on all three of us, and when the pediatrician told me to stop trying to breastfeed and just focus on bottle-feeding and pumping, I was *so relieved.* This wasn't what I imagined, but it was the best thing for Riley. He wasn't gaining weight, and this clearly wasn't working for us.

The minute we stopped trying to force nursing, things got way easier. We'd wake up to feed Riley, and Daryl would give him a bottle while I pumped. I still wasn't getting a lot of milk out, though. Even with my Elvie pumps stashed in my bra I'd get maybe 150 mL a day. That was enough for one feeding, and we supplemented with formula. By month two, Riley could latch and we had the beautiful moments I'd dreamed of having, but it wouldn't last very long. Any time he latched, he'd fall asleep before he even got a full feeding, but it felt amazing. I didn't worry about him waking up hungry because I could give him a bottle of formula.

Honestly, I felt great about this. My baby was fed, and I was doing my best. It didn't even cross my mind to feel bad about it until I shared the update on TikTok and got hundreds of messages telling me I was still a good mom. Ladies, this is how deep the mom shame and guilt and judgment go: we automatically assume that someone is going to feel bad about what their body will or won't do. Why? Because we've heard people say things about us, or about other people around us. I'll never knock breastfeeding or breast milk; I think it's a straight-up magical thing that the female body does, and yes, I got jealous of the moms on

YouTube with separate freezers filled with frozen breast milk. I wanted to be pumping and lactating like a champion cow! Breastfeeding is amazing. Pumping and bottle-feeding is amazing. And for me and my baby, formula was amazing. I just know that breastfeeding didn't work for Riley and me, and formula saved our lives.

However you choose—or need—to feed your baby, the most important thing is that they're fed.

TWENTY-TWO

FOURTH-TRIMESTER CHECKLIST

If I were in charge of things, this list would be one sentence long:

Get off your feet, rest, and heal.

That's it. I firmly believe that these few months after birth need to be sacred for you and your family and that you need time and space to heal and find your flow as a family. Now, did I take that time and space? Hell no! You already know I was skipping my Tylenol and playing hostess and acting like I was the same old Meghan and then falling apart every night. And I know that rest and time off are privileges, and that the vast majority of women in America don't get any kind of paid maternity leave, let alone parental leave for the partners who could be supporting them. There's a lot wrong with that, and it makes new parenthood even harder than it already is.

So, aside from resting and healing, what else is important this trimester?

FIND YOUR MOM SQUAD

If you're lucky enough to get knocked up at the same time as all your friends, I'm very jealous. I had to go out there and actively find a mom group, and it's not always easy to find *your* moms, the kind of women you want to hang out with whether your babies are there or not. I gotta say, this is just like dating: you're going to meet a lot of people, and while they all have great qualities and are a perfect match for *someone*, that doesn't mean they're the right match for you. Those early months can be really lonely and isolating, and the pandemic meant I couldn't just take Riley to a baby yoga class; but if you can, do it. Meet as many moms as you can, and be open to moms you might not expect. LOL, this sounds exactly like dating advice, doesn't it?

One of my favorite moms is literally almost ten years older than me and she's my ride or die. I want at least four kids and she's one and done, but I know I can text her for advice or to tell her something crazy and she won't bat an eye.

Even if you have the best partner in the world, you're going to need a support system outside of your family. I have an amazing group of moms now that I adore, and I love knowing that Riley and I have a little circle of friends to go through these milestones with. I have major anxiety, so I know it can be nerve-racking to put yourself out there, but it's worth it. Go find your moms, mama.

PLAN YOUR WORK LIFE

You and your partner already talked through your plans for work before the baby arrived, and you've already done all the paperwork with HR and your insurance company. If you're going back to your job, you should have an official start date in the calendar, and it's going to start feeling really real. Here are some things to consider:

- If the idea of starting back at 100 percent on a Monday morning feels like a lot, ask your manager about having your first day back be a Wednesday or a Thursday so you can ease into your new routine and take some of the pressure off. If your routine is going to include a childcare pickup or drop-off, do a trial run the week before so you can get a feel for what that will add to your daily commute.

- If your childcare center, babysitter, or nanny is open to it, having a trial run for your baby before you go back to work can also help ease you into this new version of life together and work out any kinks. Remember that you *and* your baby are brand-new to this experience. Ask as many questions as you want, and don't let anyone make you feel dumb or silly for it.

- Every childcare center has a whole list of guidelines: what they provide versus what you provide, what you need to bring for your baby every day, and what the designated drop-off and pickup protocols are. Review it with your partner and make sure you're both clear on everything. It can be a lot.

- All parenting is collaboration. Get really clear on what your tasks and schedules will look like when you are back at work. Who is handling pickup and drop-off? Who is the first call if the nanny or childcare center needs to contact a parent? Who will be packing up the baby bag in the morning and unpacking it at night? The little things easily feel really big, and clear communication goes a long way.

If you're staying home with your new baby, let me be clear: this is work too. No matter who does it, this is more than a full-time job and deserves all the respect in the world. And like any job, you're going to need a break from it sometimes. You'll hear more about how Daryl stepped into this role in the next chapter, but the most important thing I've heard from stay-at-home parents is that they need a break too. Being a stay-at-home parent shouldn't mean that 100 percent of the parenting duties are 100 percent your own. That's unrealistic and unfair and a recipe for burnout. If the fourth trimester feels unbalanced and you need more support, talk about it with your partner. Give them specific examples of ways they can help you and the baby and make your life feel more manageable. If you don't know where to start with this, there's a system called Fair Play developed by Eve Rodsky that makes this conversation easy and visual by turning household tasks into a deck of cards that can be divided in a way that best suits your family and your needs. The point is you cannot (and should not have to!) do it all.

TWENTY-THREE

SUPERWOMAN

I wanted to get on stage and sing for you
I wanted to start a family
I wanted to buy a house in Malibu
But there's only one of me
And I can't do it all
Call me superwoman but I know I'm not that strong
Because I cry more than a little
And if I'm superwoman
I'm flying in the rain
And I wonder will it ever get old
Being a superwoman
Smiling through the pain
Even heroes cry
So why can't I
Why can't I

— "Superwoman," from my album *Takin' It Back*

Growing up, I watched my mother do it all. She ran errands and ran a business with my dad. She was a boss and the boss of our family. She made motherhood look fun and easy, but I know my brothers and I weren't always angels (we were worse when we actually got along). I thought I'd be the twenty-first-century version of her: I'd push this baby out and come back to my old life better than ever. I planned to take three months off after Riley arrived and then get back to writing music and performing. I'd be me, just with a baby by my side. I'd planned to take off a "full" maternity leave of as many months as I could pull off before I got back to work, and two months in, the three of us were hitting our stride. We'd made it through all the nursing stress and were finally in a good groove.

Then the phone rang. It was a huge opportunity: hosting *Top Chef Family Style*. It would be six weeks of filming full ten-hour days . . . and they started in three weeks. Riley wouldn't even be three months old, and this was way sooner than I expected to go back to work. I say this knowing that the parental leave situation in America is total trash and I'm blessed to have been able to take off any time at all. And I also say this as a person who works in entertainment, where turning something down could mean the end of your career. No matter how busy or stressful things get, my team and I always say, "We're booked and we're blessed." We *are*. I *am*.

The job wasn't a matter of life or death, I know, but it was a huge opportunity, especially since I want to be on more TV shows so I can have a local, consistent job and not travel so much. And plenty of moms go back to work a whole lot earlier because they don't have a choice. This was a chance to do something I love—hosting TV—on a great show. And I could bring the baby. Daryl and Riley could be on set with me so I could get plenty of baby time while I did my job. I was scared, but our queen Oprah always says to do things that scare you . . . so I said yes.

The filming experience was so great. Everyone on that show was a joy to work with, and the time flew by. Almost everyone working on that show was a woman and a mom. One girl was even five months pregnant. I didn't even realize because she was tiny, but it made sense later why she was sitting down every day. But I still felt guilty as hell the whole time. I wasn't spending enough time with my baby. I wasn't being a good mom. All kinds of messed-up thoughts went through my head, and when I told Daryl, he'd be like, "Wait, really? You feel like that?" To everyone else, I was doing a great job. I was killing it, just like my mom had done.

But here's the thing: my mom never felt like she was killing it. She had three babies back-to-back-to-back while running a business with my dad, and she felt the same way I did: torn between her work and her family. My mom brought Ryan to work with her at the jewelry store every day for the first year of his life. He'd nap in the apartment above the store, and she'd play with him in the back while they were making jewelry and in between seeing customers. When I came along, she brought *both* of us to a day care! I always thought my mom had it all figured out, that she was Superwoman. It didn't occur to me that anyone would see *me* that way, but when you're famous and you have a baby, you get asked to do interviews and photo shoots. When people asked me about motherhood, they were saying things that didn't make any sense to me:

"You're killing it. You're amazing."

"You're always so happy and so confident."

"How do you do it all? You're Superwoman!"

I'd always get a little weird during these interviews, like, *Me? You think* I'm *doing a good job?* Because I sure as hell didn't feel like I was. How was I doing it all? Well, I was really struggling. When "All About That Bass" came out, people wanted to know how I got so confident and learned to love myself. But I don't walk around feeling confident and sure of myself all the time; I write the songs I write to remind me of what's inside me. I didn't write music to become a pop idol; I wrote songs that I needed to hear when I was a chubby, awkward thirteen-year-old who didn't think in a million years she'd grow up and have babies with the cutie from *Spy Kids*. And when *Top Chef Family Style* wrapped and it was time to write music again, what came out of me was what I needed to hear as a new mom. I poured my heart out writing "Superwoman" because it's the truth: I can't do it all.

The minute I saw Riley, I told Daryl I wanted another baby. I think I actually said, "We have to have like four more." He's used to me saying crazy shit, but I meant it. I wanted more kids right away, and I still want more kids, but I'm not sure how or when to do it. The more I wrote, the more obvious it was that the theme of the album was about feeling it *all*: the joy of a life you love, and the pain of falling short of your own expectations.

I'm lost
I'm not myself
and I wouldn't mind being anybody else
And sometimes it's hard
being covered in scars
I've run out of shooting stars
and wishing never helps
And my thoughts stay running, running
The heartbreaks keep coming, coming
Somebody tell me that I'll be okay
Come and find me
Help me put all this behind me
'cause all that I need is inside me
And only your love can remind me
—"Remind Me," from my album *Takin' It Back*

It's all there in the music: my stretch marks, my anxiety, the way that Daryl and Riley can pull me back to reality when I start to spiral.

I lugged Riley and all his baby stuff into different studios until the recording studio in our house was done. The songs were pouring out of me, and even though I could be in the same house as our baby while I was working, the guilt continued tapping on my shoulder. Daryl would bring Riley downstairs for "baby breaks" every few hours, and we'd turn down the loud music and play with him. The producers loved it, and I made sure we were done by six every day so I could be present for bath time and bedtime. And then I'd doze off while rocking him to sleep from being so exhausted and cry to Daryl about how I was a bad mom and I was never around.

"Babe," he'd say, "you're literally in the house with us all day. You're a great mom." But no matter what I did, it just never felt like enough. Being Riley's mom is the best job in the world, and loving him is so easy. But trying to be *me* and a mom, and make all the pieces fit together like they used to? That was hard.

Becoming a mama is a huge life transition, and sometimes I look at my baby and think, *I have a baby? But* I'm *a baby!* My mom says she feels the same way, and she's a fifty-three-year-old grandma. My therapist once told me that my inner child is always with me, and I feel that. I might be someone's mom, but somewhere inside me is still the awkward teenager writing songs in her bedroom about trying to love herself. Right alongside her are the versions of me I was before I met Daryl, and before we met Riley. Becoming a mom doesn't erase who we were, but it does mean we need to do some rearranging to make room for who we're becoming. Until I started freaking out about being a bad mom, I had no idea that my mom had ever felt how I feel. While I was seeing her as Superwoman, she was feeling guilty dragging us along to work and feeling guilty when she left us with a babysitter. She felt overwhelmed having three little kids so close together and spent all her extra time making sure every little thing was even among the three of us because someone (me) kept insisting that she loved the boys more.

It was never easy for my mom; it just looked that way to us kids.

Sometimes I worry that I'm making it look too easy too. So what can I do? Write a song about it.

Don't I make it look easy baby
When I do what I do
Don't I make it look easy baby
I'm fooling you
I just posted a picture
Read all the comments
Only the good ones
If I'm being honest
I might've spent an hour on it
You won't ever see me cry
'cause I've got a filter for every single lie
—"Don't I Make It Look Easy," from my album *Takin' It Back*

I'm not saying this to freak you out and tell you you're supposed to stay home with your baby. If that's what you want to do and your family can afford it, amazing, awesome, do it, and I support you. But if you're a woman who cares about her career, who really *loves* what she does, and who also really loves her baby? The balancing act can sometimes feel impossible. And from all the mamas I've met, the idea of balance seems to be bullshit. If anything, there's a sliding scale, and sometimes you're focused on your family and sometimes you're focused on your work, and no matter where your attention is, it can feel like it *should* be somewhere else. Nobody is as hard on a mother as she is on herself.

The first time I played the album for my label, I was expecting the same feedback that labels always give: "Sounds good—keep working on it!" That's the way it goes: they listen, and you go back to the studio. When we pressed Play on "Superwoman," I watched everyone's faces nervously. It's a different kind of song than I usually write. It's stripped down, bare, and heartbreaking. But when it was over, the head of my label pulled me in for a hug. "It's amazing," she said. "You've never sounded better."

We left the room that day with five songs that everyone loved, songs that came from my heart and from my first year of being a mama, songs that couldn't have existed without Daryl and Riley, without that C-section, without those bloody nipples (sorry!). Songs that I could only write from this amazing, chaotic, beautiful experience we call *motherhood*.

DEAR NEW MAMA

Dear New Mama,

I see you. The messy bun. The leggings that have just a *little* puke on them. The sore shoulders. The full heart that sometimes feels like it could break from all the love it's holding. I see you on the sleepless nights and the slow, perfect mornings. I see you on the days when you think, "*Wait, I'm a mom? Are you sure I can do this?!*"

You can. You are. You are doing it and doing it like only you can, and if you ever feel yourself slipping down a rabbit hole of comparison while you're on Instagram, stop and come back to this page. Nobody has it all figured out. Nobody has the perfect life. A lot of people are cropping out the real shit and filtering it out.

We're only at the beginning of this road, and there's so much more to come. I'm learning to live with the uncertainty and to find beauty in the in-between of it all. Whatever motherhood brings you, I hope that you know you're worthy and capable, beautiful and strong (your husband isn't lying to you, I promise). I wish you a strong support network and a partner willing to change your diaper. I wish you a healthy pregnancy and a healthy baby. I wish you a magical skin-to-skin hour with your beautiful baby. I wish you strong nipples and long naps and boobies overflowing with breast milk.

You got this, mama! I'm right here with you. It's not always easy, and it's not always gonna be cute, but it is always, always worth it.

With love, your bestie,

ACKNOWLEDGMENTS

It's hard to find people in your life who want to help you and help spread your message. Never did I ever think I would be able to write a real book. But I have to thank the queen herself, Nora McInerny, for taking my vomited notes and turning them into full, beautiful sentences. Thank you for doing all the research and spending hours writing out all these facts and bullet points that will hopefully help so many mamas-to-be out there. Thank you for your kind heart and to your brilliant mind for making me look so good. I worship you. You are an angel among us.

Thank you to Kristy Morrell, Rebecca Stanton, and Dr. Karyn Solky for sharing your knowledge and expertise with all of us anxious mamas-to-be. You are three queens who changed my life for the better, and I am forever grateful and honored to know you all.

Thank you to my managers, Tommy, Sali, Pepe, and Jeffery, for convincing me that I could pull this off and for making time for this in my chaotic schedule.

Thank you to my agent, Cait Hoyt at CAA, who helped build this baller team and make this book a reality.

Thank you to Meaghan Porter, Matt Baugher, and everyone at HarperCollins for believing in this book since day one.

Thank you to my mom for loving the shit out of me and for showing me what an amazing mother looks like. Thank you to my family and friends, my brothers, and my dad for always supporting my crazy dreams.

Thank you to my husband for ordering me dinner and taking care of our son while I wrote and edited this book for hours. But also thank you for being my number one fan and for loving me so hard. I love you too much.

And most importantly, thank you to my sweet baby boy, Riley, for teaching me patience and love at a level I didn't know was possible.

NOTES

Chapter 1: Let's Get Pregnant

1. Patricio C. Gargollo, "Male Masturbation: Does Frequency Affect Male Fertility?" Mayo Clinic, November 12, 2020, https://www.mayoclinic .org/diseases-conditions/male-infertility/expert-answers/male -masturbation/faq-20058426.
2. "How to Get Pregnant," Mayo Clinic, December 11, 2021, https://www .mayoclinic.org/healthy-lifestyle/getting-pregnant/in-depth/how-to -get-pregnant/art-20047611.

Chapter 2: Pre-pregnancy Checklist

1. "Fact Sheet #28: The Family and Medical Leave Act," U.S. Department of Labor, accessed October 13, 2022, https://www.dol.gov/agencies/whd /fact-sheets/28-fmla.
2. "Understanding the Difference Between Short-Term Disability and FMLA Leave," Thomson Reuters Legal, March 11, 2022, https://legal .thomsonreuters.com/en/insights/articles/short-term-disability-and-fmla.
3. "Pregnancy Discrimination and Pregnancy-Related Disability Discrimination," U.S. Equal Employment Opportunity Commission, accessed October 13, 2022, https://www.eeoc.gov/pregnancy -discrimination.

4. "The Benefits of Midwives," American Pregnancy Association, accessed October 13, 2022, https://americanpregnancy.org/healthy -pregnancy/labor-and-birth/midwives/.

Chapter 3: I'm Pregnant (I Think)

1. "Symptoms of Pregnancy: What Happens First," Mayo Clinic, December 3, 2021, https://www.mayoclinic.org/healthy-lifestyle /getting-pregnant/in-depth/symptoms-of-pregnancy/art-20043853.
2. "Miscarriage," Medline Plus, accessed October 13, 2022, https://medlineplus.gov/ency/article/001488.htm.

Chapter 4: First-Trimester Food and Fitness

1. "Foods to Avoid When Pregnant," American Pregnancy Association, accessed October 13, 2022, https://americanpregnancy.org/healthy -pregnancy/pregnancy-health-wellness/foods-to-avoid-during-pregnancy/.

Chapter 5: The Hard Stuff

1. Mayo Clinic Staff, "Miscarriage," Mayo Clinic, October 16, 2021, https://www.mayoclinic.org/diseases-conditions/pregnancy-loss -miscarriage/symptoms-causes/syc-20354298.
2. "Symptoms & Signs of Miscarriage," American Pregnancy Association, accessed October 13, 2022, https://americanpregnancy.org/getting -pregnant/pregnancy-loss/signs-of-miscarriage/.
3. "Miscarriage," Medline Plus, accessed October 13, 2022, https:// medlineplus.gov/ency/article/001488.htm.
4. "FAQs," American Pregnancy Association, accessed October 13, 2022, https://americanpregnancy.org/faqs/.
5. "Symptoms & Signs of Miscarriage," American Pregnancy Association.
6. "FAQs: Evaluating Infertility," The American College of Obstetricians and Gynecologists, January 2020, https://www.acog.org/womens -health/faqs/evaluating-infertility.
7. "Intrauterine Insemination (IUI)," Mayo Clinic, September 3, 2021, https://www.mayoclinic.org/tests-procedures/intrauterine-insemination /about/pac-20384722.
8. Meghan Trainor and Ryan Trainor, "Workin' on Addiction with Dr. Drew," August 3, 2022, in *Workin' on It*, produced by Lemonada

Media, podcast, MP3 audio, https://podcasts.apple.com/us/podcast
/workin-on-addiction-with-dr-drew/id1654800427?i=1000586329655.

Chapter 7: Mental Health Is Health
1. "Depression During Pregnancy," American Pregnancy Association,
   accessed October 13, 2022, https://americanpregnancy.org/healthy
   -pregnancy/pregnancy-health-wellness/depression-during-pregnancy/.
2. "Does the Affordable Care Act Cover Individuals with Mental Health
   Problems?" U.S. Department of Health and Human Services, accessed
   October 13, 2022, https://www.hhs.gov/answers/health-insurance-reform/
   does-the-aca-cover-individuals-with-mental-health-problems/index.html.

Chapter 8: Body Talk
1. "Best Sleeping Positions During Pregnancy," American Pregnancy
   Association, accessed November 16, 2022, https://americanpregnancy
   .org/healthy-pregnancy/pregnancy-health-wellness/sleeping-positions
   -while-pregnant/.
2. "Stretch Marks: Why They Appear and How to Get Rid of Them,"
   American Academy of Dermatology Association, accessed October 13,
   2022, https://www.aad.org/public/cosmetic/scars-stretch-marks/stretch
   -marks-why-appear.

Chapter 11: I Failed
1. "Gestational Diabetes," American Pregnancy Association, accessed
   October 13, 2022, https://americanpregnancy.org/healthy-pregnancy
   /pregnancy-complications/gestational-diabetes/.
2. "Gestational Diabetes," American Pregnancy Association.

Chapter 12: Second-Trimester Checklist
1. Jane Thier, "The Cost of Childcare Has Risen by 41% During the
   Pandemic with Families Spending Up to 20% of Their Salaries,"
   Fortune, January 28, 2022, https://fortune.com/2022/01/28/the-cost
   -of-child-care-in-the-us-is-rising/.

Chapter 14: Third-Trimester Checklist
1. "Top 10 Baby Names of 2021," Social Security Administration,
   accessed October 13, 2022, https://www.ssa.gov/oact/babynames/.

Chapter 18: It's Not Over . . . It's Just Beginning

1. Saba Mughal, Yusra Azhar, and Waquar Siddiqui, "Postpartum Depression," StatPearls, updated October 7, 2022, https://www.ncbi.nlm .nih.gov/books/NBK519070/.

Chapter 21: Fed Is Best

1. Erica H. Anstey, Ginny Kincaid, "Breastfeeding for Cancer Prevention," Centers for Disease Control and Prevention, August 1, 2019, https://blogs.cdc.gov/cancer/2019/08/01/breastfeeding-for-cancer -prevention/; "Breastfeeding and Diabetes," American Diabetes Association, accessed October 14, 2022, https://diabetes.org/diabetes /gestational-diabetes/diabetes-breastfeeding; Kozeta Miliku and Meghan B. Azad, "Breastfeeding and the Developmental Origins of Asthma: Current Evidence, Possible Mechanisms, and Future Research Priorities," *Nutrients* 10, no. 8 (July 2018): 995, https://doi.org/10.3390 /nu10080995; https://www.ncbi.nlm.nih.gov/pmc/articles/PMC6115903/; Liang Wang et al., "Breastfeeding Reduces Childhood Obesity Risks," *Childhood Obesity* 13, no. 3 (June 2017): 197–204, https://doi.org /10.1089/chi.2016.0210.

2. Ruchi S. Gupta et al., "Childhood Food Allergies: Current Diagnosis, Treatment, and Management Strategies," *Mayo Clinic Proceedings* 88, no. 5 (May 2013): 512–26: https://doi.org/10.1016/j.mayocp.2013.03.005.

ABOUT THE AUTHOR

Meghan Trainor is Riley's mom. Oh, and she's also the Grammy-award-winning singer-songwriter behind many of the songs you can't get out of your head. Meghan is known for her powerful voice and for her empowering messages on femininity, body image, and self-love. She's had chart-topping hits, sold millions of records, and built a loyal fanbase that adores her for her honesty, her humor, and her willingness to bring them along for the wild ride that is her life.